Occupational Therapy Practice Guidelines for

Adults With Serious Mental Illness

Catana Brown, PhD, OTR, FAOTA

Associate Professor
Midwestern University
College of Health Sciences
Glendale, AZ

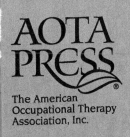

AOTA PRESS

The American
Occupational Therapy
Association, Inc.

AOTA Centennial Vision

We envision that occupational therapy is a powerful, widely recognized, science-driven, and evidence-based profession with a globally connected and diverse workforce meeting society's occupational needs.

AOTA Vision Statement

The American Occupational Therapy Association advances occupational therapy as the pre-eminent profession in promoting the health, productivity, and quality of life of individuals and society through the therapeutic application of occupation.

AOTA Mission Statement

The American Occupational Therapy Association advances the quality, availability, use, and support of occupational therapy through standard-setting, advocacy, education, and research on behalf of its members and the public.

AOTA Staff

Frederick P. Somers, *Executive Director*
Christopher M. Bluhm, *Chief Operating Officer*

Chris Davis, *Director, AOTA Press*
Ashley Hofmann, *Development/Production Editor*
Victoria Davis, *Digital/Production Editor*

Beth Ledford, *Director, Marketing*
Emily Zhang, *Technology Marketing Specialist*
Jennifer Folden, *Marketing Specialist*

The American Occupational Therapy Association, Inc.
4720 Montgomery Lane
Bethesda, MD 20814
301-652-AOTA (2682)
TDD: 800-377-8555
Fax: 301-652-7711
www.aota.org

To order: 1-877-404-AOTA (2682)

Disclaimers

This publication is designed to provide accurate and authoritative information in regard to the subject matter covered. It is sold or distributed with the understanding that the publisher is not engaged in rendering legal, accounting, or other professional service. If legal advice or other expert assistance is required, the services of a competent professional person should be sought.
—*From the Declaration of Principles jointly adopted by the American Bar Association and a Committee of Publishers and Associations*

It is the objective of the American Occupational Therapy Association to be a forum for free expression and interchange of ideas. The opinions expressed by the contributors to this work are their own and not necessarily those of the American Occupational Therapy Association.

ISBN-13: 978-1-56900-331-2
Library of Congress Control Number: 2012933474

Cover design by Jennifer Folden
Composition by Maryland Composition, Laurel, MD
Printing by Automated Graphics Systems, White Plains, MD

Contents

References 103

Figures and Tables

Acknowledgments

The series editor for this Practice Guideline is

Deborah Lieberman, MHSA, OTR/L, FAOTA
Program Director, Evidence-Based Practice
Staff Liaison to the Commission on Practice
American Occupational Therapy Association
Bethesda, MD

The issue editor for this Practice Guideline is

Marian Arbesman, PhD, OTR/L
President, ArbesIdeas, Inc.
Consultant, AOTA Evidence-Based Practice Project
Clinical Assistant Professor, Department of
　　Rehabilitation Science
State University of New York at Buffalo

The author acknowledges the following individuals
for their contributions to the evidence-based literature
review:

Dana Logsdon, MS, OTR/L
Onda Bennett, PhD, OTR/L
Robert W. Gibson, PhD, MS, OTR/L
Lynn E. Jaffe, ScD, OTR/L

Mariana D'Amico, EdD, OTR/L, BCP
Rebecca Sissom, MHSOT, OTR/L
Margarita Ortiz-Serrano, MHSOT, OTR/L
Marian Scheinholtz, MS, OTR/L.

The author acknowledges and thanks the following
individuals for their participation in the content review
and development of this publication:

Mariana D'Amico, EdD, OTR/L, BCP
Tina Champagne, OTD, OTR/L, CCAP
Christine Helfrich, PhD, OTR/L, FAOTA
Lynn Jaffe, ScD, OTR/L
Kathleen Kannenberg, MA, OTR/L, CCM
Deborah B. Pitts, PhD, OTR/L, BCMH, CPRP
Margaret (Peggy) Swarbrick, PhD, OT, CPRP
Tim Nanof, MSW
V. Judith Thomas, MGA
Madalene Palmer

The author acknowledges and thanks the following
individual for her participation in the content development of a case description:

Linda T. Learnard, OTR/L

Introduction

Purpose and Use of This Publication

Practice guidelines have been widely developed in response to the health care reform movement in the United States. Such guidelines can be a useful tool for improving the quality of health care, enhancing consumer satisfaction, promoting appropriate use of services, and reducing costs. The American Occupational Therapy Association (AOTA), which represents the interests of 140,000 occupational therapists, occupational therapy assistants, and students of occupational therapy, is committed to providing information to support decision making that promotes high-quality health care as well as wellness and educational systems that are affordable and accessible to all.

Using an evidence-based perspective and key concepts from the *Occupational Therapy Practice Framework: Domain and Process* (AOTA, 2008b), this guideline provides an overview of the occupational therapy process for adults with serious mental illness. It defines the occupational therapy domain, process, and intervention that occur within the boundaries of acceptable practice. This guideline does not discuss all possible methods of care, and although it does recommend some specific methods of care, each individual occupational therapist must make the ultimate judgment regarding the appropriateness of a given procedure in light of a specific client's circumstances and needs.

It is AOTA's intention, through this publication, to help occupational therapists and occupational therapy assistants, as well as individuals who manage, reimburse, or set policy regarding occupational therapy services, understand the contribution of occupational therapy to the provision of services to adults with serious mental

illness. This guideline also can serve as a reference for consumers, consumer providers, mental health program administrators and other mental health program staff, mental health advocates, health care regulators, third-party payers, and managed care organizations. This document may be used in any of the following ways:

- To assist occupational therapists and occupational therapy assistants in communicating about their services to external audiences
- To assist other health care practitioners, teachers, and program administrators in determining whether referral for occupational therapy services would be appropriate
- To assist third-party payers in understanding the medical necessity for occupational therapy services for adults with serious mental illness
- To assist legislators, third-party payers, and administrators in understanding the professional education, training, and skills of occupational therapists and occupational therapy assistants (see Appendix A)
- To assist program developers, administrators, legislators, and third-party payers in understanding the scope of occupational therapy services
- To assist program evaluators and policy analysts in determining outcome measures for analyzing the effectiveness of occupational therapy intervention
- To assist policy and health care benefit analysts in understanding the appropriateness of occupational therapy services for adults with serious mental illness
- To assist occupational therapy educators in designing appropriate curricula that incorporate the role of occupational therapy with adults with serious mental illness.

The first sections of this guideline include a brief discussion of the domain and process of occupational therapy. This discussion is followed by a detailed description of the occupational therapy process for adults with serious mental illness. This includes sections on referral, evaluation, and intervention. The "Intervention" section includes descriptions of occupational therapy interventions, followed by the available evidence for practice. Appendix B contains a description of evidence-based practice as it relates to occupational therapy and the process used to conduct the evidence-based reviews related to adults with serious mental illness. All studies identified in this review, including those not specifically described in the text, are summarized in the evidence tables in Appendix C. Finally, the appendixes contain additional information for occupational therapists and occupational therapy assistants relating to adults with serious mental illness, as well as examples of billing coding for occupational therapy services and other resources related to this topic.

Domain and Process of Occupational Therapy

Occupational therapy practitioners'[1] expertise lies in their knowledge of occupation and of how engaging in occupations can be used to improve human performance and ameliorate the effects of disease and disability (AOTA, 2008b).

In 2002, the AOTA Representative Assembly adopted the *Occupational Therapy Practice Framework: Domain and Process*. Informed by the previous *Uniform Terminology for Occupational Therapy* (AOTA, 1979, 1989, 1994) and the World Health Organization's (WHO's; 2001) *International Classification of*

Functioning, Disability, and Health, the *Framework* outlines the profession's domain and the process of service delivery within this domain. In 2008, the *Framework* was updated as part of the standard 5-year review cycle (AOTA, 2008b). The revisions included in the second edition focused on refining the document to reflect language and concepts relevant to current and emerging occupational therapy practice.

Domain

A profession's *domain* articulates its members' sphere of knowledge, societal contribution, and intellectual or scientific activity. The occupational therapy profession's domain centers on helping others participate in daily life activities. The broad term that the profession uses to describe daily life activities is *occupation*. As outlined in the *Framework*, occupational therapists and occupational therapy assistants[2] work collaboratively with clients to support health and participation through engagement in occupation (see Figure 1). This overarching mission circumscribes the profession's domain and emphasizes the important ways in which environmental and life circumstances influence the manner in which people carry out their occupations. Key aspects of the domain of occupational therapy are defined in Figure 2.

Process

Many professions use the process of evaluating, intervening, and targeting outcomes that is outlined in the *Framework*. Occupational therapy's application of this process is made unique, however, by its focus on occupation (see Figure 3). The process of occupational therapy service delivery begins with the *occupational profile*, an assessment of the client's occupational needs, problems, and concerns, and the

---

[1]When the term *occupational therapy practitioner* is used in this document, it refers to both occupational therapists and occupational therapy assistants (AOTA, 2006).

[2]Occupational therapists are responsible for all aspects of occupational therapy service delivery and are accountable for the safety and effectiveness of the occupational therapy service delivery process. Occupational therapy assistants deliver occupational therapy services under the supervision of and in partnership with an occupational therapist (AOTA, 2009).

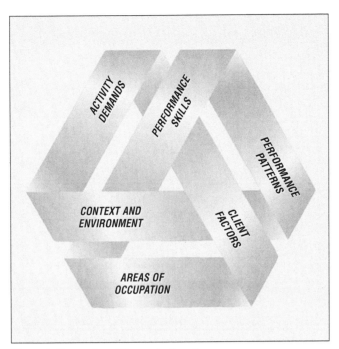

Figure 1. Occupational therapy's domain.

Reprinted from "Occupational Therapy Practice Framework: Domain and Process" (2nd ed., p. 627), by American Occupational Therapy Association, 2008, *American Journal of Occupational Therapy, 62,* 625–683. Used with permission.

AREAS OF OCCUPATION	CLIENT FACTORS	PERFORMANCE SKILLS	PERFORMANCE PATTERNS	CONTEXT AND ENVIRONMENT	ACTIVITY DEMANDS
Activities of Daily Living (ADL)*	Values, Beliefs, and Spirituality	Sensory Perceptual Skills	Habits	Cultural	Objects Used and Their Properties
Instrumental Activities of Daily Living (IADL)	Body Functions	Motor and Praxis Skills	Routines	Personal	Space Demands
Rest and Sleep	Body Structures	Emotional Regulation Skills	Roles	Physical	Social Demands
Education		Cognitive Skills	Rituals	Social	Sequencing and Timing
Work		Communication and Social Skills		Temporal	Required Actions
Play				Virtual	Required Body Functions
Leisure					Required Body Structures
Social Participation					
*Also referred to as *basic activities of daily living (BADL)* or *personal activities of daily living (PADL).*					

Figure 2. Aspects of occupational therapy's domain.

Reprinted from "Occupational Therapy Practice Framework: Domain and Process" (2nd ed., p. 628), by American Occupational Therapy Association, 2008, *American Journal of Occupational Therapy, 62,* 625–683. Used with permission.

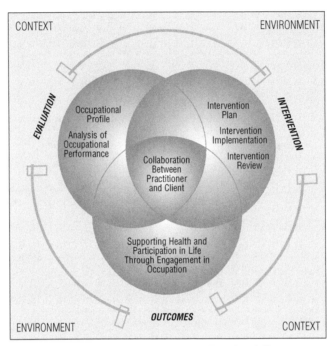

Figure 3. Occupational therapy's process of service delivery as applied within the profession's domain.

Reprinted from "Occupational Therapy Practice Framework: Domain and Process" (2nd ed., p. 627). American Occupational Therapy Association, (2008), *American Journal of Occupational Therapy, 62,* 625–683. Used with permission.

analysis of occupational performance, which includes the skills, patterns, contexts, activity demands, and client factors that contribute to or impede the client's satisfaction with his or her ability to engage in valued daily life activities. Therapists then plan and implement intervention using a variety of approaches and methods in which occupation is both the mean and end (Trombly, 1995). Occupational therapists continually assess the effectiveness of the intervention

they provide and the client's progress toward targeted outcomes. The *intervention review* informs decisions to continue or discontinue intervention and to make referrals to other agencies or professionals. Therapists select outcome measures that are valid; reliable; and appropriately sensitive to the client's occupational performance, adaptation, health and wellness, prevention, quality of life, role competence, self-advocacy, and occupational justice.

Overview of Adults With Serious Mental Illness

Background

Approximately 26% of adult Americans have a mental illness; however, the greatest burden is carried by the approximately 6% of the Americans who can be diagnosed with a serious mental illness (National Institute of Mental Health [NIMH], 2010), who are the topic of this practice guideline. The leading cause of disability in the United States is serious mental illness. For example, individuals with serious mental illness are the disability group least likely to be working, with unemployment estimates ranging between 32% and 62%, depending on the study (Cook, 2006).

Defining serious mental illness is challenging and has political, economic, and social ramifications. Definitions differ in both the clinical and policy literature; however, definitions are typically based on a combination of diagnosis, functional impairment, and duration of illness. One of the earliest definitions was provided by the National Institute of Mental Health in 1987. This definition of *severe* mental illness required that the individual have a nonorganic psychosis or personality disorder with a duration of at least 2 years and functional impairment. The Alcohol, Drug Abuse and Mental Health Reorganization Act (SAMHSA, 1993, P. L. 103-321) required the development of an operational definition of serious mental illness to be determined by the Substance Abuse Mental Health Services Administration (SAMHSA; Epstein, Barker, Vorburger, & Murtha, 2002). SAMHSA convened a group of technical experts who defined an *individual with a serious mental illness* as

> A person who is: (1) age 18 and over and (2) who currently has, or at any time during the past year had a diagnosable mental behavioral or emotional disorder of sufficient duration to meet diagnostic criteria specified within [*Diagnostic and Statistical Manual of Mental Disorders, 4th ed., text rev.; DSM–IV;* American Psychiatric Association, 2000)] or their [*International Classification of Diseases, Ninth Revision, Clinical Modification; ICD–9–CM]* equivalent (and subsequent revisions) with the exception of *DSM–IV* "V" codes, substance use disorders, and developmental disorders, which are excluded, unless they co-occur with another diagnosable serious mental illness. (SAMHSA, 1993, pp. 29,422–29,425, italics added)

A SAMHSA advisory group suggested that the term *serious impairment* be defined as impairment equivalent to a Global Assessment of Functioning (GAF) score of less than 60 (Endicott, Spitzer, Fleiss, & Cohen, 1976). GAF scores are based on clinical judgment with guidelines or examples for each 10 points, such that a score of 91–100 is indicative of superior functioning in a wide range of activities, 51–60 indicates moderate difficulty in social occupational or school functioning, and 0–10 represents a persistent inability to maintain minimal personal hygiene. In another definition, used by the Preadmission Screening and Resident Review (PASRR) to identify individuals with serious mental illness in nursing homes, any mental disorder, excluding dementia, can be classified as a serious mental illness if it results in significant functional impairment (Linkins, Lucca, Housman, & Smith, 2006). In addition, serious mental illness typically is used to determine whether mental health parity laws apply (Peck & Scheffler, 2002). Broadly speaking, *mental health parity* requires that insurance companies have equal coverage for physical and mental disorders. Three different terms are used in state parity legislation: *broad-based mental illness, serious mental illness,* and *biologically based mental illness.* Broad-based mental illness is the most inclusive term and includes all disorders listed in the *DSM–IV.* Ten states use the term *broad-based mental illness,* but 4 of those states exclude particular diagnoses, generally childhood disorders such as learning disabilities and substance abuse. Most other states use the more narrow terms *serious mental illness* and *biologically based mental illness,* in which the most commonly covered diagnoses include schizophrenia/schizoaffective disorder, bipolar disorder, major depressive disorder, obsessive–compulsive disorder, and panic disorder.

Although the specifics may vary regarding application of the definitions of serious mental illness, some aspect of the guidelines and assessment methods described typically are used by states and mental health agencies to determine who is eligible for services.

Mental Illness Diagnoses Typically Considered Serious

There is great variability in the individual impact that a psychiatric diagnosis may have on functioning, and diagnosis alone is less predictive of functional outcomes than are factors such as severity of symptomatology (Bottlender, Strauss, & Möller, 2010) and contextual issues such as financial concerns and social support (Bybee, Mowbray, Oyserman, & Lewandowski, 2003). Nevertheless, particular diagnoses are more likely to result in significant impairment in occupational performance and are more likely to be included in definitions of serious mental illness when diagnoses are specified.

Schizophrenia/schizoaffective disorder is universally considered a serious mental illness because it results in the highest levels of disability of any of the mental disorders (Ali, 2009). A diagnosis of schizophrenia requires a period of psychotic symptoms, such as hallucinations and delusions, and/or disorganized symptoms, such as thought disorder. Schizophrenia is generally accompanied by negative symptoms, such as flat affect, social withdrawal, and avolition (difficulty initiating activity). Although the positive symptoms of psychosis and disorganization typify the disorder, it is the negative symptoms that have a greater impact on functioning (Mileu, Ho, Arnd, & Andreason, 2005). Although cognitive impairment is not included in the diagnostic criteria for schizophrenia, a vast body of research indicates that cognitive impairment is both highly prevalent in schizophrenia and a strong predictor of poor outcomes (Tandon, Nasrallah, & Keshavan, 2009). Schizoaffective disorder includes disturbances in mood and can be either manic or depressive in nature.

Bipolar disorder is a mood disorder characterized by manic episodes and may or may not include depressive episodes. During manic episodes, individuals experience elevated moods; high levels of energy during which they require little sleep; pressured speech; impulsive behaviors; and, in some cases, grandiose delusions (APA, 2000). Problems in functioning (e.g., unemployment) are common in bipolar disorder, even during remission, and have been associated with degrees of cognitive impairment (Sanchez-Moreno et al., 2009).

Major depression also referred to as *unipolar depression;* its diagnosis requires that depressive episodes occur in the absence of manic episodes. Depressive episodes are typified by a depressed mood; disturbances in sleeping and eating; a lack of interest in pleasurable activities; and, at times, suicidal thoughts (APA, 2000). Although psychotic symptoms may occur, they are less common than in schizophrenia or bipolar disorder. Also, unlike people with schizophrenia and bipolar disorder, individuals with major depression are more likely to experience significant improvements in social functioning when acute symptoms are in remission (Furukawa et al., 2010).

It is important to note that serious mental illness may co-occur with other conditions, such as substance dependence, trauma, and/or personality disorders. In such cases, the serious mental illness should not be treated in isolation; instead, the occupational therapist should use a holistic and comprehensive approach that considers other relevant practice models.

Recovery Perspective: Key Components

Best practices for people with serious mental illness operate from a recovery perspective. As stated in the New Freedom Commission on Mental Health (2003),

> After a year of study, and after reviewing research and testimony, the Commission finds that recovery from mental illness is now a real possibility. The promise of the New Freedom Initiative—a life in the community for everyone—can be realized. (p. 1)

In 2004, SAMHSA convened a panel of providers, consumers, families, advocates, and others to define mental health recovery. They identified 10 fundamental components:

1. *Self-direction*—The person with mental illness should be the primary decision maker in his or her care and life.
2. *Individual and person-centered*—Each person's experience of recovery is unique.
3. *Empowerment*—The person with mental illness gains control over his or her own destiny and influences the contextual features that impact his or her life.
4. *Holistic*—Recovery involves all aspects of the person's life, including the physical, mental, and spiritual.
5. *Nonlinear*—Recovery is not a straightforward process but includes setbacks that often result in positive learning experiences.
6. *Strengths-based*—Recovery is not impairment-focused but instead capitalizes on the individual's strengths.

7. *Peer support*—Individuals in recovery benefit from the mutual social support of peers.
8. *Respect*—Individuals with mental illness should be accepted and appreciated, and self-acceptance should be fostered.
9. *Responsibility*—Individuals with mental illness are responsible for their own lives.
10. *Hope*—Recovery recognizes the potential of the individual and the vision of a positive future of full community participation.

These principles are consistent with client-centered, occupation-based occupational therapy practice. Occupational therapy practitioners strive to support individuals so they can maximize their potential and live full lives in their communities of choice. At the same time, some aspects of recovery—such as abdicating control of the therapy process and honoring the right and potential learning that occurs from making mistakes in life—may be uncomfortable for the occupational therapy practitioner; however, those aspects of recovery that cause the most discomfort can be the very components that most convey respect for the individual and his or her choices and truly promote empowerment. True empowerment means that individuals with serious mental illness are the primary decision makers in their treatment and their lives. For example, occupational therapy practitioners do not advocate smoking, but in a situation in which an individual in recovery chooses to smoke while receiving occupational therapy services to assist with money management, the occupational therapy intervention may include assistance with how to use coupons or make product selections to reduce spending on cigarettes.

Occupation-based practice is consistent with recovery's emphasis on community participation. This practice guideline and the research questions used to critically appraise the literature are most relevant for community-based practice, in which occupational therapists can best address participation in areas of occupation such as work, school, and community living. This does not exclude the role of occupational therapy practitioners in inpatient settings. For example, occupational therapists have been involved in the development of sensory-processing strategies to reduce the use of seclusion and restraint (Champagne & Stromberg, 2004). In a document published by the National Association of State Mental Health Program Directors (Huckshorn, 2005), sensory rooms were recognized as a core strategy to reduce the use of seclusion and restraint. Many existing documents and Internet resources provide additional guidance for the implementation of recovery-oriented practices (see Appendix D).

Occupational Therapy Process for Adults With Serious Mental Illness

The process of occupational therapy services for adults with serious mental illness includes evaluation and intervention focused on salient outcomes that include, but are not limited to, the individual's occupational performance, adaptation, health and wellness, participation in the community, quality of life, role competence, self-advocacy, and occupational justice (AOTA, 2008b). Although occupational therapy services often target client factors and contexts, the ultimate outcome is performance in areas of occupation. Services are initiated when an individual client's functional difficulties impede engagement in occupations and participation in everyday life activities. The evaluation includes gathering, interpreting, and synthesizing information relevant to the client's past and current occupational engagement and performance, as well as desired future participation and specific evaluation of current occupational performance.

Occupational therapy intervention is individually designed and is aimed at improving the client's desired and expected occupational engagement and participation through implementation of inventions and procedures directed at the client, the activity, and the environment. When developing an intervention, occupational therapy practitioners always consider the dynamic nature of the context and environment in which the client is expected to perform. The occupational therapy process also includes monitoring the client's response to the intervention, reevaluating and modifying the intervention plan, and measuring intervention success through outcomes that are relevant and meaningful to the individual.

The occupational therapy process is holistic and client- and family-centered, with consideration for the dynamic interaction of the individual's skills and abilities within his or her real-world environments. Occupational therapy is fluid, dynamic, and interactive, using engagement in occupations as both the method and desired outcome of the process (see the "Intervention Process" section).

Referral

The origin of the referral for occupational therapy services will vary and often depends on the setting. The attending psychiatrist is the referral source in inpatient settings such as state hospitals, Veteran's Administration (VA) hospitals, private psychiatric hospitals, forensic hospitals, and general hospitals with a psychiatric unit. In community-based settings, referrals can originate from many sources, including case managers, nurses, and rehabilitation or employment counselors. In many community settings, the client may self-refer. Common community-based settings include community mental health centers, clubhouses, community support programs, consumer-run organizations, and supported employment/housing/education programs.

A referral may be initiated with the expectation that an occupational therapy evaluation is conducted and followed by direct services. Alternatively, the referral may be consultative in nature, requiring an evaluation with recommendations for other providers. For example, the occupational therapist may receive a referral in a supported employment program, in which the therapist makes recommendations to the rehabilitation counselor, job coach, and/or employer for particular job accommodations.

Evaluation

Occupational Profile

The purpose of the occupational profile is to determine who the client is, identify the client's needs or concerns, and ascertain how these concerns affect the client's engagement in occupational performance. Information for the occupational profile is gathered through formal and informal interviews with the client and significant others. Conversations with the client help the occupational therapist gain perspective of how the client spends his or her time; what activities the client wants or needs to do; and how the environment in which the client lives, works, and socializes supports or hinders occupational engagement. The process of creating an occupational profile is fluid and evolves over time. As the occupational therapist gathers additional information during subsequent assessment and intervention sessions, the occupational profile is updated and expanded. Developing the occupational profile involves the following steps:

- *Identify the client.*
- *Determine why the client is seeking services.* Through interviews or checklists, the occupational therapist helps the client identify the current concerns relative to the areas of occupation and performance. This is a critical part of the evaluation and may be revisited throughout the recovery process as the client gains greater insight and experiences physical and cognitive changes, resulting in a new or different request for focused intervention. Assessments such as the Canadian Occupational Performance Measure (COPM; Law et al., 1998) may be helpful in setting client-centered goals for occupational performance (Jenkinson, Ownsworth, & Shum, 2007; Phipps & Richardson, 2007; Trombly, Radomski, & Davis, 1998). Administration of the COPM and similar measures requires strong interview skills. Individuals with serious mental illness may have difficulty communicating their needs and/ or be hesitant to share personal information. Creating the occupational profile requires that the occupational therapist use active listening skills. Consistent with a recovery perspective, the occupational therapist should convey a sense of respect for and appreciation of the individual as an expert on his or her own situation.
- *Identify the areas of occupation that are successful and the areas that are causing problems or risks.* On the basis of the client's concerns, goals, and aspirations, the occupational therapist identifies possible motor, cognitive, and behavioral impairments and environmental barriers and supports related to occupational performance.
- *Discuss significant aspects of the client's occupational history.* Significant aspects can include life experiences (e.g., medical interventions, employment history, vocational preferences), occupational roles, interests, and previous patterns of engagement in occupations that provide meaning to the client's life. These experiences may shape how the person deals with everyday routines and occupations. The Occupational Performance History Interview–II (OPHI–II; Kielhofner et al., 2004) is a tool that can provide information about the client's occupational history. The OPHI–II includes an extensive list of questions (with possible variations and probes) that addresses the client's occupational life history and a life history narrative. The measure includes a quantitative scoring system and a qualitative description of the life history. Ennals and Fossey (2007) found the OPHI–II to be useful in enhancing client-centered, occupation-based practice for mental health case management.
- *Determine the client's priorities and desired outcomes.* At various points in the provision of occupational therapy services, the occupational therapist and the client and/or family will discuss and prioritize outcomes so that the therapist's evaluation and intervention will match the client's/ family's desired outcomes. Truly understanding the person is a process that evolves over time. The occupational therapist continues to gather information throughout the occupational therapy process. Furthermore, observing the person in the

real environments in which he or she performs important occupations can contribute rich data to enhance the occupational profile. Tools such as the Volitional Questionnaire (Chern, Kielhofner, de las Heras, & Magalhaes, 1996) are useful for structuring the observation process and can provide data for individuals who find verbal communication challenging. In other instances, creative media, such as poetry, artwork, or photography, can contribute to the evaluation. For example, the occupational therapist might ask the client to draw a picture that depicts the individual's hopes and dreams for the future. The occupational profile is used to determine intervention strategies that will target desired outcomes. In mental health practice, the occupational therapist typically works on a team that may include psychiatrists, vocational counselors, social workers, psychologists, and/or nurses. It is important that the occupational therapist communicate with all members of the team so that the team can determine which practitioner or practitioners are best suited to address a particular client's needs.

Analysis of Occupational Performance

The occupational therapist uses information from the occupational profile to focus on the specific areas of occupation deemed relevant to the client. The occupational profile also identifies the real-world contexts in which these occupations occur. For example, the occupational therapist observes the client as he or she performs the occupations in the natural or least restrictive environment (when possible) and notes the effectiveness of the client's performance skills (e.g., motor and praxis, sensory–perceptual, cognitive, emotional regulation, communication and social) and performance patterns (e.g., habits, routines, rituals, roles):

- Select specific assessments and evaluation methods that will identify and measure the factors related to the specific aspects of the domain that may be influencing the client's performance. These assessments may focus on the client's body structures and body functions, activity

performance, or community participation. See Table 1 for examples of selected assessments.
- Interpret the assessment data to identify what supports or hinders performance.
- Develop or refine a hypothesis regarding the client's performance (i.e., identify underlying impairments or performance skill limitations that may be influencing occupational performance in multiple areas, e.g., memory impairments affecting morning hygiene, home management activities, work activities, and social interaction).
- Develop goals in collaboration with the client, and possibly the family, that address the client's desired outcomes.
- Identify potential intervention approaches, guided by best practice and the evidence, and discuss them with the client and/or family.
- Document the evaluation process and communicate the results to the appropriate team members and community agencies.

Areas of Occupation

All areas of occupation should be considered during the assessment process for people with serious mental illness. Depression and other symptoms, such as avolition, can result in neglect of activities of daily living (ADLs; Dunlop, Manheim, Song, Lyons, & Chang, 2005). Many people develop serious mental illness during adolescence or early adulthood that can interfere with the typical acquisition of instrumental activities of daily living (IADLs; Walker, Kestler, Bollini, & Hochman, 2004); extended periods of institutionalization in hospital or group home settings also can interfere with IADL acquisition. Although often neglected in the assessment process, rest and sleep disruptions are core features of mood disorders and are frequently a problem in schizophrenia and other mental illnesses (Becker, 2006). People with serious mental illness have high rates of unemployment, yet most people want to work (Cook, 2006). Limited education can contribute to difficulty in finding desirable employment (Megivern, Pellerito, & Mowbray, 2003). Leisure

Table 1. Selected Assessments Used by Occupational Therapists With Adults With Serious Mental Illness

Assessment	Purpose
Assessments used for the occupational profile	
Canadian Occupational Performance Measure (COPM; Law et al., 1998)	Interview regarding client's satisfaction and performance on occupational performance measure
Kawa River Model (Iwama, 2005)	Culturally sensitive method of assessing person in context using a river as metaphor
Occupational Circumstances Assessment Interview Rating Scale (OCAIRS; Forsyth et al., 2005)	Interview to assess occupational adaptation
Occupational Performance History Interview–II (OPHIII; Kielhofner et al., 2004)	Interview in 5 thematic areas: occupational roles, daily routine, occupational behavior settings, activity/occupational choices, and critical life events
Assessments of areas of occupation	
Modified Interest Checklist (Kielhofner & Neville, 1983)	Identifies current and past interests in leisure activities
Kohlman Evaluation of Living Skills (KELS; Thompson, 1992)	Assesses 17 living skills using interview and simulated performance
Leisure Satisfaction Scale (Beard & Ragheb, 1980)	Identifies needs satisfied through engagement in leisure activities
Performance Assessment of Self Care Skills (PASS; Holm & Rogers, 1999)	Performance assessment of 26 ADLs and IADLs, with a home and a clinic version
Rabideau Kitchen Evaluation (Neistadt, 1992)	Assesses cooking skills and kitchen safety examining 40 steps of simple meal preparation
Test of Grocery Shopping Skills (TOGSS; Brown, Rempfer, & Hamera, 2009)	Assesses accuracy and efficiency of grocery shopping in an actual grocery store
UCSD Performance-Based Skills Assessment (UPSA; Patterson, Goldman, McKibbin, Hughs, & Jeste, 2001)	Performance assessment of household chores, communication, finance transportation, and planning leisure activities
Work Behavior Inventory (Bryson, Bell, Lysaker, & Zito, 1997)	Situational assessment that measures work behaviors in the workplace
User's Guide to Worker Role Interview (WRI; Braveman et al., 2005)	Interview and observation of a person's work competencies
Assessments of performance skills	
Adolescent/Adult Sensory Profile (Brown & Dunn, 2002)	A self-report of sensory-processing preferences, with subscales measuring sensory sensitivity, sensation avoiding, low registration, and sensation seeking
Allen Cognitive Level Test (ACL; Allen et al., 2007)	Uses a leather lacing task as a screening tool to determine cognitive level based on Allen's cognitive disabilities model
Assessment of Communication and Interaction Skills (ACIS; Forsyth, Salamy, Simon, & Kielhofner, 1998)	Observational assessment that identifies strengths and weaknesses in communication and interaction while the person carries out daily occupations
Assessment of Motor and Process Skills (AMPS; Fisher, 2001)	Assesses motor and process (thinking) skills while person is engaged in ADLs
Executive Function Performance Test (Baum, Morrison, Hahn, & Edwards, 2003)	Utilizes 4 IADLs (cooking, telephone use, medication management, and bill paying) to assess executive functioning
Loewenstein Occupational Therapy Cognitive Assessment (Katz, Itzkovich, Averbuch, & Elazar, 1989)	Assesses orientation, visual and spatial perception, visuomotor organization, and thinking operations
Multiple Errands Test (Shallice & Burgess, 1991)	Assesses executive functioning through performance of several tasks (strategy use) performed in a real-world environment: a shopping mall
Test of Everyday Attention (Robertson, Ward, Ridgeway, & Nimmo-Smith, 1994)	Assesses selective, sustained, alternating, and divided attention using 8 everyday tasks, such as searching a telephone directory
Toglia Category Assessment (Toglia, 2005)	Uses a dynamic assessment process of sorting plastic utensils according to size, color, and type to measure categorization and conceptualization
Ways of Coping Checklist, Revised (Folkman & Lazarus, 1988)	Assesses different coping styles and distinguishes between adaptive and ineffective coping methods

Table 1. Selected Assessments Used by Occupational Therapists With Adults With Serious Mental Illness *(cont.)*

Assessment	Purpose
Assessments of client factors	
Empowerment Scale (Rogers, Chamberlin, Ellison, & Crean, 1997)	Assesses 5 dimensions of empowerment: self-efficacy, power, community activism, righteous anger, and optimism
Hope Scale (Snyder et al., 1991)	Self-report of hope
Volitional Questionnaire (Chern, Kielhofner, de las Heras, & Magalhaes, 1996)	Assesses a person's motivations and the environment's impact on that motivation
Assessments of context and environment	
ETHNIC Framework (Levin, Like, & Gottlieb, 2000)	Critical questions for culturally competent assessment
Recovery Assessment Scale (O'Connell, Tondora, Evans, Croog, & Davidson, 2005)	Assesses a person's ability to address life goals, involvement, diversity of treatment options, choice, and individually tailored services
Recovery Enhancing Environment Measure (Ridgway, 2005)	Assesses factors in the setting in which the individual receives services that are related to creating an environment that supports recovery
Work Environment Scale (Moos, 1994)	Measures the match between the person and the social environment in the work setting

Note. ADLs = activities of daily living; IADLs = instrumental activities of daily living; USCD = University of California, San Diego; ETHNIC = Explanation, Treatment, Healers, Negotiate, Intervention, Collaboration.

and social participation are often limited, and people with serious mental illness frequently spend much of their time alone and engaged in passive activities (Leufstadius & Eklund, 2008).

In selecting a measure, it is important to consider the appropriate assessment method. Many assessments of areas of occupation rely on self-report or informant (e.g., caregivers or mental health professionals) ratings, which may be biased (Keefe, Poe, Walker, Kang, & Harvey, 2006). Individuals tend to underreport their own problems, and informants may not be sufficiently familiar with the daily life of an adult with a serious mental illness to provide an accurate representation. Therefore, performance-based measures potentially provide a more accurate representation of an individual's ability to actually carry out different areas of occupation (Harvey, Velligan, & Bellack, 2007); however, self-report is still an important component of the evaluation. Some aspects of community functioning (e.g., satisfaction, quality of life) require a first-person perspective, and, as discussed in the "Occupational Profile" section, a person's perception of his or her daily life is always relevant information.

Performance-based measures also may be more practical for some areas of occupation than others. For example, there are available performance measures for ADLs, IADLs, and work, although existing assessments of sleep and leisure performance are primarily self-report.

Performance Skills

The evaluation of individuals with serious mental illness includes overt and subtle factors that may affect performance. *Performance skills* are the abilities clients demonstrate in the actions they perform: "Occupational therapy practitioners observe and analyze performance skills in order to understand the transactions among underlying factors that support or hinder engagement in occupations and occupational performance" (AOTA, 2008b, p. 639). The five types of performance skills are motor and praxis, sensory–perceptual, cognitive processing, emotional regulatory, and communication and social.

Motor and praxis problems are generally of less concern for people with serious mental illness than people with physical disabilities, although subtle impairments may exist. Motor speed and dexterity in particular can be impaired (Midorikawa et al., 2008) and may affect performance in areas of occupation, such as work. On the other hand, sensory processing is a major concern of people with serious mental illness because it can potentially affect all areas of occupation. For example, there is evidence that people with schizophrenia both miss and avoid sensory stimuli (Brown, Cromwell, Filion, Dunn, & Tollefson, 2002). This sensory-processing pattern results in a lack of crucial information necessary for successful participation. For instance, an individual may overlook the need for tooth brushing because he or she does not notice an unpleasant sensation from lack of oral hygiene and may avoid this aspect of self-care because he or she finds the taste of toothpaste too intense and the brushing itself uncomfortable.

Mood and anxiety disorders are by definition illnesses of emotion regulation, and schizophrenia is associated with difficulties in reading and expressing emotions (Henry et al., 2007). Communication skills are also a common area of difficulty, in particular for people with schizophrenia. Frequently discussed within the construct of social cognition, people with schizophrenia often have difficulties with empathy and reading emotions and, in individuals with paranoia, a tendency to attribute negative intentions to others (Penn, Sanna, & Roberts, 2008). For example, individuals may miss cues that another individual is bored with a conversation or uncomfortable with the proximity of personal space.

Of all the performance skills, impairments in cognitive processing are the most consistently well-documented in people with serious mental illness. A long history of research in cognition indicates that individuals with serious mental illness have cognitive impairments that affect occupational performance even more so than the symptoms of the illness itself (Green, 2006). Conversely, there is great heterogeneity among individuals with serious mental illness, so cognitive impairments and difficulties in other performance skills should not be assumed. This means that careful assessment of specific areas of cognition (e.g., attention, memory, executive function) and other performance skills is warranted to identify particular areas of impairment and strength. Psychologists may be involved in assessing cognition in people with serious mental illness using a neuropsychological assessment approach that

tends to focus on identifying the discrete cognitive skills that are impaired. When an occupational therapist examines performance skills, the assessment approach is functional in nature, meaning that the skills are examined not in isolation but in terms of their impact on daily life. Examples include the Executive Function Performance test (Baum et al., 2003), which measures cognition in the context of IADLs, and the Allen Cognitive Level Test (Allen et al., 2007), which assesses cognition by means of a leather lacing task.

Client Factors

Client factors are the underlying abilities, values, beliefs, and spirituality; body functions; and body structures that affect the individual's occupational performance. These are affected by the presence or absence of illness, disease, deprivation, and disability. Client factors support the individual's performance skills.

Values, beliefs, and spirituality are important in supporting an individual's interest or motivation toward pursuit of a particular area of occupation. For example, an individual is more likely to pursue college coursework if he or she values education. Spirituality often is viewed as an integral component of the recovery process. Spirituality can heal the wounds associated with the lived experience of mental illness by providing meaning and a positive sense of self (Bussema & Bussema, 2007).

The term *body functions* refers to the "physiological function of body systems (including psychological functions)" (WHO, 2001, p. 10). *Body structures* are the "anatomical parts of the body" (WHO, 2001, p. 10). Body structures and body functions are interrelated (e.g., the heart and blood vessels are body structures that support cardiovascular functions, such as blood pressure). In the case of serious mental illness, occupational therapists are most likely to be interested in the body functions related to mental functioning; however, because functions such as attention and memory are very difficult to assess outside of the context of an activity, generally speaking, occupational therapists who work with people with serious mental illness are more likely to assess performance skills as opposed to body functions. On the other hand, occupational therapists may assess symptoms or self-efficacy, which could be considered a psychological body function, or components of recovery, such as hope and empowerment.

Performance Patterns

Performance patterns are "behaviors related to daily life activities that are habitual or routine" (AOTA, 2008b); they include habits, routines, rituals, and roles. Serious mental illness often results in an impoverishment of roles. Things that typically give people a sense of identity and help establish daily habits and routines of roles such as worker, parent, student, and family member can be lost to a person with a serious mental illness. Resumption of roles can lead to better well-being. One study, for example, found that individuals with mental illness who spent more time in employment had better ratings of health, wellness, and functioning than those who were not working (Eklund & Leufstadius, 2007). Occupational therapists assess current roles as well as roles that individuals have held in the past and roles they desire for the future.

In addition, during the evaluation process, occupational therapists identify habits and routines, often through an assessment of how the individual spends the day. This is important in determining how a lack of habits or an overly routinized schedule may influence an individual's occupational performance. For example, there is research that for individuals with bipolar disorder, a disruption in routines, such as the timing for sleeping and eating, can lead to the onset of manic and depressive episodes (Malkoff-Schwartz et al., 1998).

Contexts and Environments

Occupational therapists acknowledge the influence of cultural, personal, temporal, and virtual contextual factors, as well as physical and social environmental factors, on occupations and activities. Contextual and environmental factors that support or inhibit occupational performance of individuals with serious mental illness should be identified throughout the evaluation and intervention process. Stigma is a contextual factor that presents a major barrier to participation in full community functioning for people with mental illness.

Another major contextual issue for people with serious mental illness is economic, with most people with serious mental illness living below the poverty level. The social disadvantage of poverty may be a larger factor in unemployment and homelessness than the illness itself (Draine, Salzer, Culhane, & Hadley, 2002).

Activity Demands

Determining whether a client may be able to complete an activity depends not only on the individual's performance skills, performance patterns, and client factors but also on the demands the activity itself places on the person. These activity demands are aspects that include the tools needed to carry out the activity, the space and social demands required by the activity, and the required actions and performance skills needed to take part in the given activity. After the occupational therapist and client have identified relevant areas of occupation to address, it becomes necessary to identify the activity demands of those areas of occupation that are specific and unique for the client within his or her natural environment. For example, in a work setting, the occupational therapist needs to identify those activity demands that are part of the client's assigned duties, along with the work setting, materials, tools, and social requirements of the work. If money management is an identified area of occupation to be addressed, information related to income, expenses, and methods for paying bills will need to be gathered.

Occupational therapists, through their use of activity analysis, can identify the type of activity and environment in which the client can perform at his or her best. During the course of occupational therapy intervention, occupational therapy practitioners grade and vary the activity demands of the selected intervention task and the environment in which it is performed to provide the client with a "just-right challenge" that will be therapeutic without exceeding his or her current level of skills. As the client improves, the therapist gradually modifies the activities to provide more challenge to the client. Therapists assist the clients in their ability to perform under the current environment and activity demands, and therapists consider how future changes in the environment and activity may challenge the client's skill level. Part of the rehabilitation process may include training the client to identify environmental barriers to performance and how to modify the environment to improve performance (e.g., when studying, turning off the radio and beginning the most challenging topic first).

Clients with serious mental illness may need adaptive equipment and environmental modifications to engage in the selected activities (e.g., changes to the tools or utensils used in the activity, reorganization of equipment and supplies in the environment). The occupational therapist should carefully analyze the client's need for environmental modifications and adjust the modifications to the client's cognitive ability to learn new ways of approaching and completing activities.

Interpreting the Evaluation Results

The occupational therapist analyzes and synthesizes the results of the evaluation to create a picture of the strengths and resources that might be used to promote occupational performance and the barriers that prevent successful participation. These results should be documented as required by the setting but also in such a way that they are accessible and meaningful to the client and treatment team. Documentation of evaluation results typically includes a written report and also may include oral presentations in team meetings. The client always should be apprised of the evaluation results. When the family is involved, and if the client agrees, it can be helpful to include the family in the evaluation process. The occupational therapist then uses the evaluation results and information from other treatment team members to, in collaboration with the client, develop an intervention plan.

Intervention Process

Intervention Plan and Implementation

As a part of the occupational therapy process, the occupational therapist develops an intervention plan that considers the client's goals, values, and beliefs; the client's health and well-being; the client's performance skills and performance patterns; collective influence of the context, environment, activity demands, and client factors on the client's performance; and the context of service delivery in which the intervention is provided (e.g., caregiver expectations, organization's purpose, payer's requirements, applicable regulations; AOTA, 2008b). The intervention plan outlines and guides the therapist's actions and is based on the best available evidence to meet the identified outcomes (AOTA, 2008b).

Once the therapist has identified targeted goals in collaboration with the client and/or family, the therapist determines the intervention approach that is best suited to address the goals. Intervention approaches used by occupational therapy practitioners include the following:

- *Prevent,* an intervention approach designed to address clients with or without disability who are at risk for occupational performance problems (Dunn, McClain, Brown, & Youngstrom, 1998); for example, interventions to prevent self-harm for individuals with emotion regulation concerns
- *Establish and restore,* an intervention approach designed to change client variables to establish a skill or ability that has not yet developed or to restore a skill or ability that has been impaired (Dunn et al., 1998); for example, restoring cognitive skills such as memory or attention to improve work performance, or developing skills in money management
- *Modify* activity demands and the contexts in which activities are performed to support safe, independent performance of valued activities within the constraints of motor, cognitive, or perceptual limitations; for example, simplifying recipes for basic dishes the client would like to cook
- *Create or promote* a healthy and satisfying lifestyle that includes adherence to a medication routine, appropriate diet, appropriate levels of physical activity, and satisfying levels of engagement in social relationships and activities by providing enriched contextual and activity experiences that will enhance performance for all persons in the natural contexts of life (Dunn et al., 1998); for example, helping with the choice of a new apartment that will be affordable given the individual's financial

situation and in a neighborhood in which the individual can feel safe

- *Maintain* performance and health that the individual with serious mental illness has previously regained or that the psychiatric disability has spared; for example, helping the individual maintain his or her current level of physical activity by introducing him or her to others who enjoy the same activities.

Often, the intervention plan in the client's record is developed by members of the team with input from the occupational therapist. This intervention plan may be fairly general and not specify the specific approaches and objectives for the occupational therapy intervention. In this case, it is important that the occupational therapist

documents an occupational therapy plan of care and, in collaboration with the client, specifies the goals and occupational therapy intervention approaches.

See Table 2 for examples of interventions used with adults with serious mental illness organized according to the approaches identified above. Occupational therapy practitioners also should consider the types of interventions when determining the most effective treatment plan for a given client. The types of interventions include therapeutic use of self; therapeutic use of occupations and activities, which includes preparatory methods, purposeful activity, and occupation-based activity; consultation; and education. Although all types of occupational therapy interventions are used for all approaches, therapeutic use of

Table 2. Intervention Approaches and Examples of Occupation-Based Goals for Adults With Serious Mental Illness

Approach	Intervention Focus	Intervention Examples
Restore/remediate: Designed to change client variables to establish a skill or ability that has been impaired (Dunn McClain, Brown, & Youngstrom, 1998)	Performance skills	Cognitive rehabilitation to support work performance
	Performance patterns	Establish regular schedule for going to bed and getting up in the morning to improve sleep hygiene
	Occupation	Teach skills for using public transportation
Modify, compensate, adapt: Designed to find ways to revise the task, method, or environment to support performance (Dunn et al., 1998)	Occupation	Use alarm system or phone to provide alert to take medication
	Context	Educate coworkers on mental illness to reduce stigma in the workplace
	Activity demands	Utilize automatic bill pay service to improve money management
Maintain: Designed to provide the supports that will preserve the performance capabilities clients have regained so they can continue to meet their occupational needs	Performance skills	Make sure that social skills taught are utilized regularly in the natural environment
	Performance patterns	Create a household cleaning calendar that can be updated by the client
	Occupation	Have case manager continue to provide feedback and support for IADLs skills taught by occupational therapist
	Context	During apartment search, identify neighborhood with sidewalks so that client can address the need for physical activity
	Activity demands	Ensure that job placement is a good match for person's skills and abilities
Prevent: Designed to prevent performance problems by supporting body structures and functions, performance skills environment, and habits and routines (Dunn et al., 1998)	Performance skills	Teach stress management to prevent relapse and anxiety that interferes with occupational performance
	Performance patterns	Recommend that the individual schedule shopping for less busy times, to reduce environmental pressures
	Context	Ensure that inpatient services do not use seclusion or restraints to prevent trauma associated with those procedures
	Activity demands	Allow for breaks during class time to prevent overload
Create/promote: Does not assume a disability is present or any factors interfere with performance; designed to provide enriched contextual and activity experiences that enhance performance for all persons in the natural contexts (Dunn et al., 1998)	Performance patterns	Provide services at times that match typical performance patterns (e.g., work during day; leisure on nights and weekends)
	Context	Provide culturally sensitive interventions
	Activity demands	Create opportunities for strengths to be recognized and for client to engage in activities in which they contribute to others

Note. IADLs = instrumental activities of daily living.

self (i.e., therapist's use of his or her personality, perception, and judgment; AOTA, 2008b) is an overarching concept that should be considered in each therapeutic interaction. Therapeutic use of self is a vital responsibility of the occupational therapist and occupational therapy assistant, as well as all members of the health care team.

Intervention Review and Outcome Monitoring

Intervention review is a continuous process of reevaluating and reviewing the intervention plan, the effectiveness of service delivery, and progress toward targeted outcomes (AOTA, 2008b). Reevaluation may involve readministering assessments or tests that were used at the time of initial evaluation, having the client complete a satisfaction questionnaire, or answering questions to evaluate each goal. Reevaluation substantiates progress toward goal attainment; indicates any change in functional status; and directs modifications to the intervention plan, if necessary (Moyers & Dale, 2007).

Discontinuation, Discharge Planning, and Follow-Up

Like all components of the occupational therapy process, the client should be involved in decisions related to discontinuation, discharge planning, and follow-up. Oftentimes, services for people with serious mental illness are provided in community-based mental health settings, which generally do not have strict limitations for occupational therapy in terms of length of stay or number of visits. Services typically are discontinued when progress is no longer being made, goals are achieved, or the client makes a decision to discontinue occupational therapy. Regardless of the reason for discontinuation of services, it is important that a discharge plan is developed. In some cases, another provider (e.g., a case manager) may take over monitoring and support to ensure that the client maintains his or her highest level of performance. The occupational therapist also may schedule follow-up visits to reassess the status of the client and determine whether occupational therapy services should be reinstated. Occupational therapy services may be reinitiated if the client needs a refresher to retain skills or new concerns are identified by the client or therapist.

Reimbursement, Documentation, and Billing

Coverage and payment for occupational therapy services provided for persons with severe mental health diagnoses vary greatly, depending on setting and payer policies. Inpatient mental health services and those that are paid as a bundled rate for multiple program services (e.g., community mental health day programs) are more likely to be covered under traditional medical insurance. Private insurance companies often subcontract mental health reimbursement to specialized companies that do not recognize occupational therapists as approved mental health practitioners, with resulting denials for any occupational therapy claims for mental health diagnoses. In addition, recognition of specific *Current Procedural Terminology™ (CPT)* codes (American Medical Association, 2011) varies by payer; therefore, it is important for therapists and providers to communicate with individual payers about their specific coverage and payment rules governing both occupational therapy and mental health diagnoses.

Assuming that the payer will cover mental health services provided by occupational therapists under the client's policy, the most important factor in ensuring claims approval is effective documentation.

Occupational therapy practitioners carefully document their services in the areas of evaluation, intervention, and outcomes (AOTA, 2010). They also document their recommendations and communicate them to the other team members and the client. This documentation should be completed "within the time frames, format, and standards established by the practice settings, agencies, external accreditations programs, payers, and AOTA documents" (AOTA, 2010, p. S109).

The purpose of occupational therapy documentation is to
- "Articulate the rationale for the provision of occupational therapy services and the relationship of this service to the client's outcomes
- Reflect the therapist's clinical reasoning and professional judgment

- Communicate information about the client from an occupational therapy perspective
- Create a chronological record of client status, occupational therapy services provided, and client outcomes." (AOTA, 2008a, p. 684)

The following types of documentation may be completed for each client, as mandated by legal requirements, the practice setting, third-party payers, or some combination of these (AOTA, 2008a):

- Evaluation or screening report
- Occupational therapy service contacts
- Occupational therapy intervention plan
- Progress report
- Prescription or recommendation for adaptive equipment
- Reevaluation report
- Discharge or discontinuation report.

Documentation must disclose all sources of information that were used to formulate the conclusions (assessment tools, methods, observations, client's perceptions and feedback, family input). AOTA's (2008a) "Guidelines for Documentation of Occupational Therapy" outline specific report contents and fundamental elements of documentation.

Appendix E identifies the *CPT* codes, with descriptions and examples that occupational therapists use when billing for services.

Specific Interventions and Related Evidence

The following sections include both an overview of specific interventions and findings from the systematic reviews of occupational therapy for adults with serious mental illness. A standard process of searching for and reviewing literature related to practice with adults with serious mental illness was used and is summarized in Appendix B. All studies identified by the reviews, including those not specifically described in this section, are summarized and cited in full in the evidence tables in Appendix C. Readers are encouraged to read the full articles for more details. Most of the interventions reviewed focus on areas of occupation and include interventions that target education, work, community living, and health and wellness. In addition, there is a significant body of evidence related to interventions that target cognition using either a remediation or compensation approach.

Education

Many individuals with serious mental illness are *undereducated,* meaning they have not achieved their desired level of education. Oftentimes, the onset of illness in early adulthood has interfered with their completion of higher education goals. Limited education can have far-reaching effects that influence self-esteem and desired employment. A qualitative study of individuals with psychiatric disabilities who had participated in higher education found that barriers to successful completion included symptoms and hospitalizations that made it difficult to concentrate, complete assignments, and memorize material; financial concerns; and the social isolation often associated with stigma (Megivern et al., 2003). In addition, these individuals rarely disclosed their mental illness or sought out student services.

Interventions are needed to help individuals with serious mental illness succeed in higher education. Educational goals include completing a general equivalency diploma (GED), obtaining a technical training certificate, taking adult education courses at a community college, or attaining a college degree. It is only recently that interventions specifically targeting adult education have been developed, with supported education being the most widely accepted approach.

Supported Education

The goal of supported education is to assist individuals with serious mental illness in meeting their postsecondary education goals (Mowbray et al., 2005). Many principles of supported education grew out of the previously developed supported-employment programs. In supported employment (discussed in more detail shortly), there is an emphasis on choice and immediate placement in real work settings with appropriate supports. The individual chooses the educational experience and setting, and the necessary supports are put in place so that the individual may succeed in that experience. Supported education includes interventions that target performance skills and the context. Performance skills that are addressed can include basic knowledge for educational competence (e.g., math, writing, computer skills, public speaking), stress management, time management, and social skills so that the individual can function effectively in the academic setting. Environmental supports involve accessing existing resources on campus, such as tutoring, student counseling, advising, and financial aid services, and also may include the provision of additional supports, such as education/assistance with rights related to reasonable accommodations for people with psychiatric disabilities. Different models of supported education exist, with some programs provided on campus and others taking place at a mental health setting, such as a clubhouse.

Evidence for Supported Education

Two Level I studies examined the efficacy of supported education. In the first study, a randomized controlled trial, the Bridge Program was compared with treatment as usual at a mental health center (Gutman, Kerner, Zombek, Dulek, & Ramsey, 2009). The Bridge Program, developed by occupational therapists, is a 12-module supported-education intervention administered over 6 weeks that includes topics such as time management, study skills, and exploration of educational/vocational interests. Of the 38 participants, 21 were assigned to the intervention group and 17 to the control group, but only 16 intervention participants completed the program. At the end of the program, 10 of the 16 participants were involved in job training, an educational program, or had obtained employment or were applying to a program, whereas only 1 control group participant was involved in coursework. Attendance was related to success in the program.

The second study was a larger randomized controlled trial conducted by Collins, Bybee, and Mowbray (1998). In this study ($N = 397$), participants were randomly assigned to one of three groups: (1) classroom-supported education with curriculum addressing managing the campus, career exploration, and stress management ($n = 135$); (2) group-supported education ($n = 134$) that explored career end education choices and assisted with use of educational resources; and (3) individual unstructured support ($n = 128$). There were no differences among the groups for outcomes related to work or school; as a whole, participants who completed the study doubled their enrollment in educational and vocational programs. Although there was a high dropout rate, individuals with higher levels of participation had better outcomes related to motivation, satisfaction, enjoyment, and learning.

Two Level III studies examined the efficacy of supported education. The first, conducted by Gutman and colleagues (2007), was a pilot of the Bridge Program just discussed. The authors used a pretest–posttest design, with 18 participants; the results indicated improvements on 10 of the 12 module posttests. Twelve participants enrolled in further coursework.

In the second study, Unger, Anthony, Sciarappa, and Rogers (1991) examined a continuing education program focused on vocational interests and competencies, along with career planning; participants developed a specific vocational goal and identified the vocational and educational skills and resources needed to attain that goal. Thirty-five of the initial 52 participants completed the 4-semester program and had increased rates of competitive employment or enrollment in an educational program after completing the program, as well as increased self-esteem and decreased levels of hospitalization.

Summary of the Evidence for Supported Education

At this time, the evidence related to supported education is limited; however, the results of existing studies are promising, in that they suggest that supported education may help individuals with serious mental illness pursue goals related to higher education. Preliminary evidence suggests that the level of engagement in the supported-education program is associated with outcomes; therefore, it is important that occupational therapists use strategies to promote attendance and active participation.

Work

People with serious mental illness have the highest unemployment rates among people with disabilities, with estimates ranging from 32% to 62% (Cook, 2006). Most people with serious mental illness express a desire to work, and those who are working report that work contributes to the recovery process (Honey, 2003; Provencher, Gregg, Mead, & Mueser, 2002). Specific benefits of work include regular involvement in meaningful activity and social relationships, along with improved mental health and self-efficacy. The development of a worker role begins for most individuals in adolescence and early adulthood; however, for many individuals with serious mental illness, this is a vulnerable time period that often is disrupted by the first episodes of their mental illnesses (Gioia, 2005). There are many other barriers to employment that people with serious mental illness must face, including discrimination, employment disincentives, and low educational attainment (Cook, 2006). Effective interventions to address high unemployment rates for individuals with serious mental illness are critically needed.

Supported Employment

Supported employment is the most studied intervention approach to promote work for people with serious mental illness. Some of the approaches in supported employment were developed in reaction to negative outcomes associated with prevocational programs (e.g., sheltered workshops), which tended to provide long-term training with little success in regard to placement in competitive employment positions. A primary innovation of supported employment is that individuals begin their job search on program entry and are placed quickly in a competitive employment position (Bond, 2004). On the job site, the employee is provided with necessary supports and training. Other key characteristics of supported employment include coordination of employment and mental health services, job placement based on the individual's preferences and goals, support provided as long as is necessary, and Social Security benefits counseling.

Evidence for Supported Employment

Three Level I systematic reviews have examined the efficacy of supported employment for people with serious mental illness. In the first, Crowther, Marshall, Bond, and Huxley (2001) reviewed randomized controlled trials that compared supported employment with prevocational training. There were three major findings: (1) Prevocational training did not result in competitive employment, (2) supported employment did promote placement in competitive employment, and (3) supported employment had superior outcomes when compared with prevocational training in terms of hours worked and income.

In the second review, Twamley, Jeste, and Lehman (2003) conducted a meta-analysis of randomized controlled trials comparing three conditions—supported employment (which included the individual placement and support [IPS] model), job-related social skills training, and Incentive Therapy (a Veterans' Administration [VA] program that offers part-time employment within the VA hospital)—with a control condition. Nine of the 11 studies in their review compared supported employment with a control, with only 1 study each for job-related social skills training and Incentive Therapy. The overall effect size for all 11 studies was .66. The effect size for the 9 studies that used supported employment was higher: .79. Despite this relatively impressive effect size, only 51% of the participants in supported employment obtained work, leaving many participants unemployed.

In the third study, Bond, Drake, and Becker (2008) reviewed the IPS model of supported employment and specifically limited the review to studies with high fidelity to the model. The 11 studies included in their review found that the employment rate for participants in the IPS condition was 61%, compared with 23% for control participants, and those in the

IPS condition obtained their first job 10 weeks earlier than control participants. Two-thirds of individuals in the IPS condition who were competitively employed worked 20 hours or more.

Many Level I randomized controlled trials have examined the efficacy of supported employment. In a large, 8-site study, 1,273 participants were randomly assigned to supported employment or to a control group of traditional vocational services (Cook, Leff, et al., 2005; Cook, Lehman, et al., 2005). Participants in the supported-employment condition had higher rates of competitive employment (55% vs. 34%), more participants worked 40 or more hours per month (51% vs. 39%), and participants' median income was higher ($122/month vs. $99/month). Individuals in programs with highly integrated psychiatric and vocational rehabilitation services were 2½ times more likely to work competitively and had more hours of work than individuals in the low-integration programs. This study was conducted over a 24-month period, with supported-employment outcomes improving over time.

In a Level I randomized controlled trial of 204 participants, Mueser and colleagues (2004) compared the IPS model of supported employment with a psychosocial rehabilitation program or standard vocational services. The IPS model was superior to the other two services for all vocational outcomes, with the exception of job satisfaction. Participants in the IPS condition had higher levels of competitive employment: 73.9% vs. 18.2% for psychosocial rehabilitation and 27.5% for standard vocational services. Participants in the IPS condition also had impressive rates of job retention over 2 years (>90%). There were few differences in nonvocational outcomes for the three groups.

Rogers, Anthony, Lyass, and Penk (2006) compared supported employment using the Choose–Get–Keep model with enhanced state vocational rehabilitation in a Level I randomized controlled trial of 135 participants. The Choose–Get–Keep model is one of the earliest programs in supported employment, and it places an emphasis on choice. The program includes both classroom instruction and individual meetings. Both programs resulted in improvements in vocational outcomes, self-esteem, and quality of life and were equally successful.

Latimer and colleagues (2006) compared supported employment ($n = 75$) with traditional vocational services ($n = 75$) in a Level I randomized controlled trial. Supported employment resulted in higher employment rates; however, there were no differences between the groups for total hours worked or earnings. This study was conducted in Canada, a country that provides greater monthly disability income than the United States, which could have contributed to the lack of differences in earnings.

Additional studies have examined the efficacy of supported employment when augmented with other services. For example, McGurk, Mueser, Feldman, Wolfe, and Pascaris (2007) studied supported employment along with the Thinking Skills for Work program in a small Level I randomized controlled trial ($N = 44$). The Thinking Skills for Work program uses computerized activities for cognitive training. Individuals in the combined program were compared with individuals in supported employment alone. The results indicated that the combined program had better outcomes than supported employment alone for finding and keeping a job, hours worked, and earnings. Other studies have investigated supported employment combined with social skills training.

Mueser and colleagues (2005) compared a combined program of social skills training and supported employment with supported employment alone in a Level I randomized controlled trial with 35 participants. There was no difference between the two groups for numbers of participants working, hours worked, or earnings, but the combined group participants had more workplace knowledge.

Tsang, Chan, Wong, and Liberman (2009) compared a combined IPS program and social skills training with IPS alone or traditional vocational rehabilitation. A total of 163 participants were randomly assigned to groups. Participants in the combined program had better vocational outcomes than those in the other programs, but there were no differences between groups for nonvocational outcomes.

Some studies of supported employment have focused on its efficacy for specific populations. In a study of older adults, Twamley and colleagues (2005) compared the IPS model with Department of Rehabilitation (DOR) employment services, which provides job preparation and development skills, and the Wellness and Vocational Enrichment (WAVE) program, which provides prevocational counseling. The IPS program was superior in terms of percentage of participants who obtained volunteer or paid work: 81% vs. 44% in the WAVE program and 29% in DOR.

Supported employment also was evaluated in a rural setting where services are more loosely linked and there may be fewer job opportunities (Gold et al., 2006). A combined Assertive Community Treatment (ACT) and IPS model was compared with traditional vocational services. The ACT–IPS model resulted in high rates of employment: 80%, compared with 38% for traditional services. The earnings were also higher for participants in ACT–IPS.

Evidence for Other Work Interventions

This section will review the efficacy of work programs other than supported employment. Tsang and Pearson (2001) examined the efficacy of work-related social skills training to help people with schizophrenia find and keep jobs. In their Level I randomized controlled trial, they assigned 97 participants to one of three groups: (1) a work-related social skills training program with follow-up contact, (2) a work-related social skills training program without follow-up, or (3) standard outpatient psychiatric care. At a 3-month follow-up, 46.7% of the participants in the social skills training group were employed, 23.1% of the participants in the social skills training group without follow-up were employed, and only 2.4% of the participants in the standard outpatient psychiatric care group were employed.

Lee, Tan, Ma, Tsai, and Liu (2006) studied the efficacy of a stress management program in individuals employed in a hospital's job program. Using Level I random assignment within a crossover design, they compared participants for the 12 weeks they received stress management with 12 weeks they did not. The program was effective in reducing stress during the intervention, but improvements were not maintained.

Three studies were conducted in a VA medical center to investigate the efficacy of work programs that place participants in positions within the VA system. In one Level I study, participants were randomly assigned to receive feedback using the Work Behavior Inventory (WBI) or usual supports (Bell, Lysaker, & Bryson, 2003). Participants in the WBI program had better job performance and worked more hours than the usual support group. Another Level I randomized controlled study using the WBI program for older adults in a VA medical center found that older adults benefited similarly to younger adults in terms of vocational outcomes (Bell, Fiszdon, Greig, & Bryson, 2005). Still another Level I randomized controlled study within the VA system using WBI feedback along with neurocognitive enhancement therapy found better outcomes for neurocognition compared with work therapy alone; however, there were few differences in vocational outcomes for the two groups (Bell, Bryson, Greig, Corcoran, & Wexler, 2001).

Kates, Nikolaou, Ballie, and Hess (1997) studied the efficacy of an in-home employment program with 52 participants using a Level II quasi-experimental design. Work tasks were brought to the client's home, with staff support provided twice a week. The work program was compared with standard outpatient care. Participants in the work program were more likely to join other work programs. While participating in the in-home program, their earnings were three times that of individuals employed in local sheltered workshops.

Evidence for Factors Related to Work Success

Identifying factors related to success in the work setting is helpful in the process of designing effective interventions. Bell and Bryson (2003) compared individuals with improved work performance with individuals who did not improve, using the WBI in a Level II cohort study. Those with improved work performance had better scores on a series of cognitive measures. Similarly, Lysaker, Bell, and Bioty (1995), using a Level III pretest–posttest design, found that cognitive impairments were associated with fewer improvements after work rehabilitation. Participants in a Level I large randomized controlled trial for supported employment (Cook et al., 2005) were studied to identify clinical factors that were associated with employment outcomes (Razzano et al., 2005). More positive symptoms (e.g., hallucinations, delusions, disorganized thinking) were associated with better employment outcomes, whereas more negative symptoms (e.g., flat affect, avolition, anhedonia) were associated with worse employment outcomes. A Level I randomized controlled trial found that training related to specific work skills was more effective than creative arts activities in teaching work tasks (Kopelowicz, Liberman, Wallace, Aguirre, & Mintz, 2006).

Summary of Evidence for Work-Related Interventions

There is substantial and strong evidence for the efficacy of supported employment in improving vocational outcomes for people with serious mental illness. There is a great deal of variability in the studies in terms of employment rates, yet large numbers of persons with serious mental illness remain unemployed even with intervention; however, programs with high fidelity to the model tend to result in greater improvements. As a whole, supported employment has its greatest impact on the number of individuals who are competitively employed, job tenure, and earnings. There is little support for benefits from supported employment related to nonvocational outcomes. Other work programs that specifically target work-related skills show promise. Additional attention is needed to address the still-high rates of unemployment for people with serious mental illness and to target individuals who tend to perform more poorly in work programs, such as those with cognitive impairments and/or negative symptoms.

Community Living

For several reasons, individuals with serious mental illness may need interventions that address community living. Some individuals may be living in their own apartments for the first time and have limited experience with money management, cooking, home management, or other IADLs necessary for indepen-

dent living. Others may have lived independently for an extended period of time but have specific goals related to improving their quality of life (e.g., socializing with others, better money management, increased involvement in leisure activities).

Skills Training

Skills-training approaches often are used to help individuals with serious mental illness develop the necessary skills for successful and satisfying community living, such as managing an apartment or taking medications as prescribed. The broad area of social skills is another common focus of skills-training programs. Individuals with serious mental illness may have challenges in communicating thoughts and feelings and interpreting the communications of others (Couture, Penn, & Roberts, 2006). As a result, impaired social skills may interfere with the development of interpersonal relationships and make it difficult to succeed in aspects of community life that require interaction, such as collaborating with health care providers or making a request of a landlord.

Skills training is based on behavioral and learning theories and involves identifying the target behaviors to be taught; breaking those behaviors down into component parts; and teaching the skills through demonstration, didactic instruction, and practice (Bellack, 2004). In addition to performing the behavior during skills training sessions, homework frequently is provided so that individuals can practice skills in their natural environments. Regular feedback and reinforcement are essential components of a skills-training approach. Most skills-training programs are conducted in groups using a module format, with each module focusing on a particular skills area. Some programs teach a wide range of community living skills (Patterson et al., 2006), whereas others focus on a specific skill, such as parenting (Phelan, Lee, Howe, & Walter, 2006) or grocery shopping (Brown, Rempfer, & Hamera, 2002).

Evidence for Skills Training

Several systematic reviews that have examined the efficacy of skills training have yielded conflicting conclusions. A meta-analysis of social skills conducted by Corrigan (1991) concluded that individuals with serious mental illness could acquire and maintain new skills, and the review found that outcomes were better in outpatient settings compared with inpatient settings. A Level I meta-analysis conducted by Dilk and Bond (1996) examined a broader range of skills, including social and prevocational skills and IADLs, and found that individuals could acquire new skills; however, there was inadequate evidence to support the generalization of a specific skill (e.g., assertiveness) to larger areas of role functioning. In addition, duration of training was related to effect size, indicating that longer programs were more effective.

In contrast, a Level I meta-analysis of social-skills training conducted by Pilling and colleagues (2002) did not find that social skills training was more beneficial than other interventions, and Robertson, Connaughton, and Nicol (1998) found inconclusive results when they compared life-skills training programs with traditional rehabilitation such as recreation, art, and occupational therapy. A Level I Cochrane review (Tungpunkom & Nicol, 2008) found no evidence to support the use of life-skills training programs. One reason for the differing conclusions could be the study selection: The studies that found less optimistic results (Pilling et al., 2002; Robertson et al., 1998; Tungpunkom & Nicol, 2008) were more stringent and specific in terms of the types of programs included, and they restricted their review to randomized controlled trials.

As a result, these reviews included only 2 to 9 studies in their analysis, whereas Dilk and Bond (1996) included 68 studies and Corrigan (1991) included 73 studies. The most recent update of the Schizophrenia Port Outcomes Research Team (PORT) recommended skills training as an evidence-based intervention for people with schizophrenia (Dixon et al., 2010). The PORT recommendation is based on a systematic review of the literature, along with an analysis by an expert panel.

Numerous Level I studies support the efficacy of skills training as an intervention for people with serious mental illness. In some cases, multiple studies have examined the efficacy of a specific skills-training program. For example, the Functional Adaptation Skills Training (FAST) program—a manualized group intervention addressing medication management, social skills, communication skills, organization and planning, transportation, and financial management—has been studied in three randomized controlled trials (Patterson et al., 2003, 2005, 2006). A study that compared FAST with an attention control group addressing personal problems found that participants in the FAST program improved more on everyday living skills and social skills compared with the control group, but there was no difference in symptom improvement (Patterson et al., 2006). A study of FAST with older adults found greater improvements in everyday living skills when compared with a treatment-as-usual control group (Patterson et al., 2003). The FAST program was adapted for a Latino population and named Program for Training and Development of Skills in Latinos (PEDAL; Patterson et al., 2005). In a study that compared PEDAL with a time-equivalent support group, the PEDAL group improved more than the control group in everyday functioning, but not in social skills.

Another program studied in several Level I randomized controlled trials is the University of California, Los Angeles (UCLA) Social and Independent Living Skills Program. The manualized UCLA program has modules related to basic conversation, recreation for leisure, medication management, and symptom management. In one of the earliest studies, the UCLA skills training program was compared with supportive group therapy (Marder et al., 1996). Modest improvements in social functioning were found for skills training, and outcomes were most favorable when social skills training was combined with a low-dose medication regimen. In a study that compared the UCLA program with crafts-based occupational therapy, Liberman and colleagues (1998) found that the skills training group improved more than the occupational therapy group in the areas of living skills, self-esteem, and distress. The skills training program was very intensive, meeting 3 hours a day, 4 days a week, for 6 months. The differences between the groups found at 6 months were no longer significant at the 12- and 24-month follow-ups. A brief form of the UCLA modules, with 16 sessions of 45 minutes each, also was compared with occupational therapy (Kopelowicz, Wallace, & Zarate, 1998). Participants in the skills-training program had better scores than participants in the crafts-based occupational therapy group on a knowledge and performance test focused on the skills taught in the skills training program.

To address concerns related to declines at follow-up and generalizability to real life, Glynn and colleagues (2002) developed the In Vivo Amplified Skills Training (IVAST), which combines the UCLA modules with intensive case management. The case manager supports the skills training by creating opportunities to apply the skills in natural environments and by establishing support systems to maintain the use of those skills. In a study comparing IVAST to traditional skills training, IVAST resulted in better and quicker skills acquisition (Glynn et al., 2002).

The UCLA modules have been adapted for several populations. The modules were examined in a Latino population in a Level I randomized controlled trial; the results indicated greater improvements in symptoms and skill acquisition when compared with a group that received customary outpatient care (Kopelowicz, Zarate, Gonzalez Smith, Mintz, & Liberman, 2003). Improvements in functioning were not maintained at follow-up.

Anzai and colleagues (2002) adapted the brief version of the UCLA program for Japanese persons and studied it by comparing skills training with conventional occupational therapy that consisted of crafts, reality orientation, and work assignments. The skills-training program resulted in greater improvements on the living skills measure compared with crafts-based occupational therapy.

In an adaptation for outpatients in Spain, Moriana, Alarcon, and Herruzo (2006) modified the UCLA modules for individual in-home use. This Level II non-randomized controlled trial examined only outcomes related to symptoms (not skill acquisition) as measured by the Positive and Negative Syndrome Scale (PANSS; Kay, Fisbein & Opler, 1987) and found that the intervention group had lower scores when compared with participants who received conventional treatment.

The efficacy of other skills-training interventions also have been supported with Level I randomized controlled trials. In a study of a 48-week psycho-social skills–training group for individuals from Mexico, the results indicated better outcomes in the areas of symptoms and psychosocial functioning when compared with a treatment-as-usual control group (Valencia, Rascon, Juarez, & Murow, 2007). In an occupational therapy study, verbal versus experiential forms of money management skills training were compared (Bickes, DeLoache, Dicer, & Miller, 2001). This short intervention of only 2 weeks resulted in improvements for both groups on the Comprehensive Occupational Therapy Evaluation (COTE) scale (Brayman, Kirby, Misenheimer & Short, 1976) and no improvements on the Milwaukee Evaluation of Daily Living Skills (Leonardelli, 1988). No differences between groups were detected.

Duncombe (2004), an occupational therapist, specifically examined the effects of context on the skills training experience for people with schizophrenia. Participants were randomly assigned to learn cooking in either a clinic situation or their home. Both groups improved significantly on their cooking skills, but the setting in which the training took place did not affect the outcomes. In another study, the researchers used a board game to teach social skills to people with schizophrenia (Torres, Mendez, Merino, & Moran, 2002). Participants were randomized to one of three groups: (1) the social skills board game, psychomotor skills training, and motor activities–based occupational therapy; (2) social-skills training without the board game, psychomotor skills training, and motor activities–based occupational therapy; or (3) motor activities–based occupational therapy. More improvements in social skills were noted for participants in the first group, which included the board game.

Choi and Kwon's (2006) study of social cognition enhancement training (SCET) included 36 sessions focused on social cognition and problem solving. They compared SCET with standard psychiatric rehabilitation and found that better outcomes were associated with SCET. They also found that some skills required 6 months of intervention before change occurred.

In a study that combined social skills training with cognitive–behavioral approaches, Granholm and colleagues (2005) noted that the intervention group had a reduction in positive symptoms and engaged in more social functioning than the control group, but their level of performance did not improve.

Level II studies in which nonrandomized groups are compared and Level III single group pretest–posttest designs also have found primarily positive outcomes for skills training:

- In a Level II nonrandomized study of older adults with serious mental illness, skills training plus health care management resulted in better outcomes than health care management alone (Bartels et al., 2004).
- In a study that used a coping skills module in a Level II nonrandomized controlled trial, intervention participants had better outcomes than a matched group of control participants in the areas of hygiene, self-esteem, and delusions (Leclerc, Lesage, Ricard, Lecomte, & Cyr, 2000).
- Participants in the role development program demonstrated greater improvements in social roles, task skills, and interpersonal skills when compared with participants in a multidepartmental activity program in a Level II nonrandomized controlled trial (Schindler, 2005).
- An extended skills-training intervention covering five different areas of community functioning indicated improvements in life skills and symptoms from pretest to posttest in a Level III study (Halford, Harrison, Kalyansundaram Moutrey, & Simpson, 1995).
- An activity group to improve social interaction skills was more effective than verbal discussion in a control group, as found in a Level II nonrandomized controlled trial (Schindler, 1999).
- Individuals with schizophrenia improved their grocery shopping skills from pretest to posttest after participating in a 9-session Level III grocery

shopping intervention (Brown, Rempfer, & Hamera, 2002).
- In a preliminary Level III pretest–posttest study that examined a group life-skills session focused on food and nutrition, no significant improvements were observed (Helfrich, Aviles, Badiani, Walens, & Sabol, 2006).
- Another study of the life-skills program described in the preceding item found that, contrary to prediction, participants with lower scores on the Allen Cognitive Level Screen (ACLS)–2000 (Allen, Earhart, & Blue, 1992) showed more improvement than participants with higher ACLS–2000 scores (Helfrich, Chan, & Sabol, 2011).
- A Level III pretest–posttest study of a parenting program for individuals with mental illness found improvements in parenting skills and high levels of satisfaction among the participants (Phelan et al., 2006).

Summary of Evidence for Skills Training for Community Living

Numerous studies have examined the efficacy of skills training for people with serious mental illness. As a whole, this body of research indicates that people with serious mental illness can acquire and maintain new skills. The evidence also suggests that longer, more extensive training tends to result in better outcomes. There is limited generalizability of skills, suggesting that it is important to teach the skills that are most relevant to the individual and within the situations in which he or she will apply those skills. The efficacy of skills training for improving symptoms is equivocal, with some studies indicating improvements and others not.

Health and Wellness

The relationship between physical and mental health always has been appreciated by occupational therapy practitioners, yet only recently has this relationship received much attention in regard to people with serious mental illness. Individuals with serious mental illness have high rates of physical illnesses, yet their general health condition tends to be neglected by health care providers. In addition, people with serious mental illness are more likely than the general population to engage in lifestyle behaviors that contribute to poor physical health, including sedentary lifestyles, inadequate nutrition, smoking, poor sleep, and not seeking out physical health care (Vreeland, 2007). So egregious is the health care disparity that one study found decades of potential life lost for public mental health clients in comparison to the general population in the same states (Colton & Manderscheid, 2006), with the most common cause of death being cardiovascular disease. There are many other common comorbid conditions among people with serious mental illness that could be prevented or better managed with lifestyle changes, including obesity, diabetes, osteoporosis, and poor dental health (Leucht, Burkard, Henderson, Maj, & Sartorius, 2007; Newcomer & Hennekens, 2007).

Evidence for Health and Wellness Interventions

There is no generally accepted model of intervention to address health and wellness concerns for people with serious mental illness. This is partially due to the emerging nature of this area of practice; however, the importance of psychosocial interventions to address health and wellness is receiving increasing attention. For example, the updated PORT recommendations for people with schizophrenia suggests that overweight and obese individuals with serious mental illness should attend a weight loss program of at least 3 months' duration (Dixon et al., 2010).

The systematic reviews included findings related to interventions associated with occupational therapy's domain of practice. Cabassa, Ezell, and Lewis-Fernandez's (2010) Level I systematic review of lifestyle interventions to address obesity, cardiovascular disease, and diabetes included 23 randomized and nonrandomized controlled trials (Levels I and II). They found that 12 of 23 studies reported significant improvements in weight loss or metabolic syndrome.

A Level II nonrandomized controlled trial that examined the efficacy of an intervention to improve nutrition and physical activity for weight loss found significant improvements in weight, body mass index, waist circumference, and self-reported physical activity (Brown, Goetz, Van Sciver, Sullivan, & Hamera, 2006). In a Level I randomized controlled trial, Chafetz, White, Collins-Bride, Cooper, and Nickens (2008) compared a wellness training program with standard care. The wellness program was an individualized skills-training program. Although there was a high dropout rate, participants in the wellness program had greater improvements on perceived physical function and general health status.

Another study addressed HIV infection (Weinhardt, Carey, Carey, & Verdecias, 1998). This small Level I randomized controlled trial found that assertiveness training was effective in improving assertiveness skills, HIV knowledge, and behavioral intentions for people with serious mental illness.

Approaches to address routines and engagement in meaningful activities also have found positive outcomes. Frank and colleagues (2005) used a Level I randomized controlled trial to examine the efficacy of interpersonal and social rhythm therapy (IPSRT) on time to remission for people with bipolar disorder. IPSRT focuses on lifestyle issues related to maintaining daily routines and managing disruptions to such routines. The results indicated that participants in IPSRT had a longer time before remission compared with participants who received intensive clinical management.

Edgelow and Krupa (2011) conducted a pilot study to examine the efficacy of an occupational time use intervention called "Action Over Inertia." This approach uses an individualized workbook to promote engagement in meaningful activities. A small randomized controlled trial found that intervention participants spent 47 more minutes per day in meaningful activities compared with control participants.

Several studies have examined specifically the impact of physical activity on mental health. A Level I systematic review that examined physical activity for people with depressive and anxiety disorders found that increased activity and exercise training resulted in a decrease in anxiety and depression (Dunn, Trivedi, & O'Neal, 2001). A Level I randomized controlled trial that examined the effects of exercise on depression found that a high dose of exercise was more effective than a low dose or control condition in reducing depression and remission rates (Dunn, Trivedi, Kampert, Clark, & Chambliss, 2005).

Using a Level II quasi-experimental design, Hutchinson, Skrinar, and Cross (1999) investigated the effect of aerobic exercise in adults with serious mental illness. Individuals who exercised had better self-esteem and less depression, and there was a trend toward improvement in ADL performance and satisfaction. Kelley, Coursey, and Selby (1997) used an outdoor adventure program with a Level III pretest–posttest design to investigate the impact of activities such as hiking, rock climbing, spelunking, and canoeing on function in people with serious mental illness. They found that participants had an increase in self-esteem and a decrease in depression and anxiety, as well as improvements in trust and cooperation and hostility and interpersonal sensitivity.

Although these studies are diverse in terms of the intervention approaches and outcomes studied, there is promising evidence to indicate that individuals with serious mental illness can make lifestyle changes that support health and wellness. The increased attention and concern related to physical health for people with serious mental illness suggests that much research will be published in this area in the future, which will allow for clearer guidelines related to the types of interventions that are most effective.

Cognition

Individuals with serious mental illness often experience cognitive impairments. Some cognitive impairments that are well-documented in schizophrenia include deficits in processing speed, attention, working memory, and executive function (e.g., verbal learning, problem solving, social cognition; Green, 2006). Similar impairments are core features of bipolar disorder and seem particularly prominent

in individuals with greater psychosocial dysfunction. Although cognitive impairments often are present in depression, unlike with schizophrenia and bipolar disorder, when the primary symptoms of depression are alleviated, significant improvements in cognition can be expected (Gualtieri, Johnson, & Benedict, 2006). It is important to note that there is a great deal of heterogeneity in terms of the expression of cognitive impairments; therefore, assumptions about cognitive impairments in a particular individual should not be made simply on the basis of diagnosis.

Occupational therapy practitioners should be particularly interested in this area of research, because cognitive impairments present a primary barrier for successful occupational performance in people with serious mental illness. For example, cognitive impairments in bipolar disorder interfere with successful work, family, and social life (Sanchez-Moreno et al., 2009). Lysaker and Buck (2007) suggested that there are three reasons why cognitive impairments present significant problems for people with schizophrenia: (1) Limited cognitive abilities prevent skill acquisition; (2) cognitive impairments result in an avoidant coping style, limiting one's interaction with the world and others; and (3) cognitive impairments impede the development of a coherent sense of self, such that individuals with schizophrenia are less likely to persist when faced with adversity.

Cognitive Remediation

Cognitive remediation is used as an intervention approach with the belief that by ameliorating basic cognitive deficits, individuals with serious mental illness are better able to participate in daily life and are more capable of acquiring new skills. Cognitive remediation is based on models of *neuroplasticity*, which suggest that neural processes are enhanced by engaging in activities that target specific cognitive functions (Kern, Glynn, Horan, & Marder, 2009). Computers or pencil-and-paper tasks typically are used to target specific areas of cognitive impairments. Activities are graded, and once mastery is achieved, individuals move on to exercises that are more cognitively complex.

Evidence for Cognitive Remediation

Three Level I systematic reviews and a Level I meta-analysis examined the efficacy of cognitive remediation in people with serious mental illness. Pilling and colleagues (2002) indicated that cognitive remediation is not effective in improving basic cognitive functions in schizophrenia. In their systematic review of three studies, McGrath and Hayes (2000) suggested that there is no conclusive evidence supporting cognitive remediation for people with schizophrenia. Another small review of three studies that specifically examined problem-solving training did not support the efficacy of cognitive remediation (Xia & Li, 2007).

On the other hand, a meta-analysis that examined both improvements on trained tasks and generalization to psychosocial functioning found significant improvements, with medium effect sizes for cognitive performance and psychosocial functioning (McGurk, Twamley, Sitzer, McHugo, & Mueser, 2007). In addition, this study found that results were better for psychosocial functioning when cognitive remediation was paired with psychiatric rehabilitation. The difference in findings may be due to study selection, with those reviews that did not find support for cognitive remediation having stricter inclusion criteria.

For the most part, Level I randomized controlled trials provide support for improvement on cognitive tests with differing findings related to functioning. One study conducted by occupational therapists compared an instrumental enrichment (IE) intervention that targeted cognitive impairments with traditional occupational therapy that used functional tasks and expressive activities (Hadas-Lidor, Katz, Tyano, & Weizman, 2001). The results indicated better outcomes on the cognitive tasks for the IE group, which also had greater improvements in work and residence status with no difference on IADLs and self-concept.

A study of the Neurocognitive Training Program (NCR) found benefits for the cognitive remediation group as compared to the control participants on some, but not all, measures (Wykes, Reeder, Corner, Williams, & Everitt, 1999). NCR participants demonstrated better self-esteem, cognitive flexibility, and memory. Wykes and colleagues (2003) examined the long-term effects of cognitive remediation and found that improvements in memory lasted the longest.

Two Level I randomized controlled studies compared computer-assisted cognitive remediation with another computer-based intervention without cognitive-specific challenges. One study found that both groups improved in all areas of cognition assessed (working memory, verbal episodic memory, spatial episodic memory, processing speed, and reasoning; Kurtz, Seltzer, Shagan, Thime, & Wexler, 2007). Working memory was the only area in which the cognitive remediation group improved more than the computer control group, suggesting that the use of the computer may have some generalized effects on cognition.

Conversely, a similar study that compared computer-based cognitive remediation with a computer control group found that participants in the cognitive remediation group had better outcomes than the computer control group in overall cognitive functioning, psychomotor speed, and verbal learning (Lindenmayer et al., 2008). There was no difference between the two groups in terms of work functioning or symptoms.

Integrated psychological treatment (IPT) combines cognitive remediation and skills training. In a pretest–posttest design, IPT was beneficial in the areas of symptoms, cognitive and social functioning, and quality of life (Briand et al., 2006). In a Level II nonrandomized controlled trial, Roder and colleagues (2002) examined cognitive remediation in the context of social skills training. Four groups were compared; three were considered intervention groups that investigated a problem-solving training program within the context of a residential, vocational, or recreational setting, and the fourth, the control group, used IPT. All groups had improvements in psychosocial functioning, with the control group experiencing greater relapse.

Cognitive Adaptation Training

Another approach to addressing cognitive impairments in people with serious mental illness is to adapt the environment to compensate for those impairments. Velligan and colleagues (2000, 2006) developed a manualized approach to modifying the environment called *cognitive adaptation training*. Occupational therapists were involved in the development of this model, contributing to both the assessment and the intervention components. In cognitive adaptation training, individuals with serious mental illness first are assessed to determine the nature of their cognitive impairment. In one study (Velligan et al., 2000), Allen's Cognitive Levels test was included in the cognitive assessment, then environmental supports or modifications were put into place to simplify the cognitive demands. For example, closets and cabinets are organized; checklists are developed for specific ADLs or IADLs; or signs are used to remind the individual to lock the door, turn off the oven, or take the keys when leaving the house.

Evidence for Cognitive Adaptation Training

Two Level I randomized controlled trials have examined the efficacy of cognitive adaptation training. In the initial study, with a total of 45 participants in 3 groups (cognitive adaptation training, an attention control group, and a standard medication follow-up group), participants in the cognitive adaptation training had better outcomes than the other 2 groups in symptom levels, adaptive functioning, and relapse (Velligan et al., 2000). A slightly larger randomized controlled trial with 60 participants in 2 groups specifically examined the clients' use of the available supports (Velligan et al., 2006). One group received cognitive adaptation training and the other received generic adaptations such as alarm clocks and calendars with the expectation that the individual set up their own support. The results indicated that individuals in the cognitive adaptation program were much more likely to use the available supports.

Errorless Learning

Another way to compensate for cognitive impairments is to alter the method of instruction. *Errorless*

learning is a method of teaching that attempts to eliminate mistakes in the learning process (Terrace, 1963). The theory is that when mistakes are made while learning, the error information becomes encoded in memory. When the individual attempts to retrieve a memory, the wrong information interferes with the retrieval of the correct information. Errorless learning thereby prevents the encoding of the wrong information.

In errorless learning, repeated practice typically is used in a manner such that the learner is not allowed to guess or try out a skill until it is clear that the correct information has been encoded. Errorless learning has been applied to many populations with cognitive impairments, including individuals with schizophrenia (Kern, Liberman, Kopelwicz, Mintz, & Green, 2002; O'Carrol, Russell, Lawrie, & Johnstone, 1999).

Evidence for Errorless Learning

In a Level II study, individuals with schizophrenia were divided into 2 groups: individuals with and without memory impairment (O'Carrol et al., 1999). The results indicated that individuals remembered more words when using an errorless learning approach as opposed to learning that allowed for mistakes. In addition, the participants with memory impairments received more benefit from errorless learning, suggesting that that this approach worked by compensating for cognitive deficits.

Further support for errorless learning was provided by Kern and colleagues (2002), who used the approach—specifically, two entry-level job tasks—to teach functional skills to people with schizophrenias. This Level I study found that individuals who practiced errorless learning had better outcomes than individuals who received conventional instruction. In addition, a secondary analysis suggested that errorless learning compensated for cognitive deficits, particularly in the area of verbal memory (Kern, Green, Mintz, & Liberman, 2003).

Table 3. Case Descriptions: Adults With Serious Mental Illness

Patient Description	Occupational Therapy Evaluation/Reevaluation	Occupational Therapy Goals	Occupational Therapy Interventions

▪ Includes diagnosis/condition/ problem manifestation
▪ May include impairments, barriers to activities, contexts
	▪ May include
	  – Occupational profile
	  – Assessments used
	  – Clinical observations
		▪ Should include only the goals addressed by the occupational therapist, not other members of team or other professionals	▪ Should include only what the occupational therapist does that requires the skills of the occupational therapist
			▪ Descriptions should include wording such as "*The occupational therapist develops, trains, recommends, instructs, etc.*"

Cara, age 25, and would like to return to college to finish her degree. She has a diagnosis of bipolar disorder with psychotic features. She takes lithium to stabilize her mood and aripíprazole (Abilify) to control delusions. Although her symptoms are relatively controlled, she occasionally hears voices and experiences racing thoughts, which can make it difficult to focus. Cara lives alone in an apartment that is about 5 miles from the college she would like to attend. She receives services from the community mental health center, including seeing a case manager who visits her weekly. Cara is a self-referral for the supported-education program.	▪ The occupational profile indicates that Cara attended 2 years of college before experiencing her first symptoms of mania and psychosis. She would like to complete her degree in art history and eventually get a job in an art museum. Cara is concerned about her ability to concentrate to allow her to be successful in school. She also is worried that other students and faculty will not accept her. ▪ The occupational therapist administers the Adolescent/Adult Sensory Profile (Brown & Dunn, 2002) and finds that Cara is highly sensitive to sensory stimuli, suggesting that she may become distracted in the classroom. ▪ The occupational therapist uses skilled observation during the supported-education class and indeed finds that Cara is distractible and lacks confidence.	▪ Cara will enroll in an art history course after completing the supported-education class. ▪ Cara will be able to concentrate sufficiently in her first college course as demonstrated by a passing grade on 90% of assignments and tests. ▪ Cara will identify a study partner and meet with this partner at least 3 times during the semester.	▪ The occupational therapist enrolls Cara in a supported-education class that the occupational therapist has developed and leads. Class content includes computer and study skills, making presentations, negotiating the university system, and strategies for obtaining living accommodations and improving self-confidence. ▪ Activities include role-playing to facilitate peer and teacher–advisor interaction. ▪ The occupational therapist provides one-on-one instruction to help Cara identify reasonable accommodations needed to enhance her ability to concentrate, such as sitting in the front row of class and taking tests in a separate room free from distractions. ▪ The occupational therapist recommends compensatory activities and adaptations (e.g., selecting course times when Cara is most alert, engaging in physical activity prior to class, setting a vibrating reminder on her phone to help her focus in class). ▪ The occupational therapist meets with Cara as needed to help prioritize assignments and problem-solve concerns. ▪ The occupational therapist develops a monthly group therapy session for students from the supported-education class to provide peer support and share success stories.

Table 3. Case Descriptions: Adults With Serious Mental Illness *(cont.)*

Patient Description	Occupational Therapy Evaluation/Reevaluation	Occupational Therapy Goals	Occupational Therapy Interventions
José, age 37, has expressed an interest in returning to work, although he doesn't know where to begin. José has a diagnosis of schizophrenia. He receives minimal mental health services, primarily medication. José is referred to the vocational team at the community mental health center to pursue interests in work. The team that will work with José includes a rehabilitation counselor, an occupational therapist, and a job coach.	▪ The occupational therapist completes an occupational profile that indicates that José has a limited work history. As a young adult, José worked in construction, but he has not worked since age 25. José enjoys being outside and around animals. He spends a lot of time walking around his neighborhood and knows all of the pets. He also knows many of the local shop owners and clerks. The occupational therapist incorporates information from the rehabilitation counselor's Self Directed Search (SDS; Holland, 1997) assessment that indicates José's type as realistic, investigative, and social. ▪ The occupational therapist observes José in his volunteer position. She notices that the other volunteers tend to avoid José. He tends to carry on lengthy conversations and miss social cues from his coworkers. In addition, he regularly brings up delusional material in conversation. On the other hand, the supervisor is understanding of José's talkative nature and unconventional topics of conversation. She is pleased with his ability to complete assigned tasks, his enthusiasm, and concern for the animals.	▪ José will locate and begin working in a volunteer position for at least 5 hours/week within 1 month. ▪ José will successfully complete assigned tasks in the volunteer job as reported by his supervisor with sufficient competency to continue in the position. ▪ José will reduce the delusional content of conversation to no more than 1x/day. ▪ José will carry on a reciprocal conversation with a coworker and will initiate ending the conversation when the coworker displays nonverbal signs of disinterest at least 1x/day.	▪ On the basis of the occupational profile and the SDS, the occupational therapist recommends that José begin his volunteer job search by looking for jobs that involve animals and the opportunity to socialize with others. José applies and is accepted for a volunteer position for 10 hours/week. ▪ José and the occupational therapist meet outside of work to address social relationships with José's coworkers. They discuss and make a list of topics José should avoid when talking to his coworkers. In addition, they role-play numerous scenarios between coworkers. José is taught to identify nonverbal communication and how to gracefully end a conversation. ▪ The occupational therapist consults with José's supervisor to find additional social support at work. The supervisor identifies a coworker who will likely be open to interacting with José, and the supervisor creates opportunities for the two to work side by side. ▪ After working at the animal shelter for several months, José's supervisor informs him of a paid position that involves taking care of animals over the weekend at a veterinary clinic. She acts as a reference, and José succeeds in getting the job.

(continued)

Table 3. Case Descriptions: Adults With Serious Mental Illness *(cont.)*

Patient Description	Occupational Therapy Evaluation/Reevaluation	Occupational Therapy Goals	Occupational Therapy Interventions
	■ The occupational therapist completes the Work Environment Impact Scale (Moore-Corner, Kielhofner, & Olson, 1998) to examine José's perceptions of the supports and barriers in his new position at the veterinary clinic. For the most part, José is comfortable in the new setting; however, the work is more variable, and he feels uncomfortable asking for help or clarification.	■ José will work his assigned 16 hours/week and receive adequate performance evaluations to maintain employment.	■ The occupational therapist and José meet with the assigned supervisor. The supervisor agrees to write down José's tasks for the day and review them in the morning before he begins work. In addition, José role-plays with the therapist the process of asking for help as needed. ■ The occupational therapist meets with José monthly outside of the workplace to provide support and problem-solve any evolving concerns.
Mai, age 22, with a diagnosis of major depressive disorder (MDD). She was recently admitted to the inpatient psychiatric unit of an acute care hospital after a suicide attempt. She is very guarded and shy and rarely speaks unless someone speaks to her.	■ The occupational therapist administers the Canadian Occupational Performance Measure (COPM; Law et al., 1998) as a component of the occupational profile. Mai indicates she is living away from her family for the first time and does not know anyone in her apartment complex. She feels overwhelmed with the responsibilities of living on her own and is particularly concerned about money management, for which she rates herself on performance as a 5 out 10 and on satisfaction as a 3 out of 10. ■ The Assessment of Communication and Interaction Skills (Forsyth, Salamy, Simon, & Kielhofner, 1998) indicates that Mai feels awkward in social situations. She is reluctant to initiate conversation and rarely makes eye contact. She speaks so softly that others often have to ask her to repeat herself. Some of these patterns of social interaction are related to her Asian background, and Mai reports she is more comfortable around her Asian family.	■ Mai will develop a budget that accounts for her monthly income and expenditures. ■ Mai will set up an automatic bill pay system for her rent and utilities. ■ Mai will report an increase of at least 3 points in the areas of performance and satisfaction on the COPM measure of money management. ■ Mai will initiate a conversation with peers at least 3x/day. ■ Mai will make eye contact during conversation 50% of the time during social skills role play. ■ Mai will increase her voice projection so that others ask her to repeat herself no more than 2x/day.	■ The occupational therapist works individually with Mai on money management. She instructs Mai on how to create a monthly budget. They work together to set up an online bill pay system with automatic withdrawals for rent and utilities. ■ The occupational therapist readministers the COPM to assess improvements in the area of money management. ■ Mai attends the social skills training group developed and led by the occupational therapist. The group incorporates social role play and social problem-solving situations based on real-life experiences that the group members identify as challenging. The group meets 3x/week, and group members receive homework to practice skills outside of the group sessions. ■ The occupational therapist recommends that, on discharge, Mai attend a weekly support group where she can continue to work on her social skills and potentially develop additional social supports.

Table 3. Case Descriptions: Adults With Serious Mental Illness *(cont.)*

Patient Description	Occupational Therapy Evaluation/Reevaluation	Occupational Therapy Goals	Occupational Therapy Interventions
Stanley, age 52, is facing eviction from his apartment because he is having trouble meeting the landlord's standards for home maintenance. Stanley has a diagnosis of schizophrenia. He acknowledges his difficulties with home management, and because he has been homeless in the past, he is particularly fearful of having to face that experience again. He is highly motivated to maintain his apartment, although his landlord is giving him little time to rectify the situation. Stanley receives mental health services in his home through an assertive community treatment (ACT) team.	■ The occupational therapist meets Stanley at his apartment to evaluate the situation. She finds the apartment in disarray. The occupational therapist meets with the landlord during her visit. One of the primary concerns of the landlord is that Stanley leaves food out until it becomes spoiled, and the food attracts insects that infest not only Stanley's apartment but also nearby apartments. ■ The occupational therapist administers the Performance Assessment of Self-Care Skills (PASS; Holm & Rogers, 1999). During this administration, Stanley is able to complete the different IADLs but often misses details and does not complete the task satisfactorily. For example, when sweeping the floor, he leaves quite a bit of the debris and doesn't seem to notice. ■ The occupational therapist administers the Loewenstein Occupational Therapy Cognitive Assessment (LOTCA; Katz, Itzkovich, Averbuch, & Elazar, 1989) and the Test of Everyday Attention (Robertson, Ward, Ridgeway, & Nimmo-Smith, 1994). Stanley has significant problems in all areas of attention and has difficulty with visual motor organization and problem solving. He has good memory and comprehension abilities.	■ Stanley will clean his apartment with the help of his occupational therapist so that it will pass inspection by the landlord. ■ Stanley will adequately maintain his apartment as assessed with weekly inspections from the occupational therapist.	■ To address the immediate crisis of avoiding eviction and help tackle the initial task of cleaning that is overwhelming Stanley, the occupational therapist will work with a family member on strategies for Stanley to follow to complete this home maintenance activity. In her meeting with the landlord, the occupational therapist asks for an extension to get the apartment in order, and he agrees. The occupational therapist draws up a contract with Stanley that clarifies the expectation regarding Stanley's role in the initial cleaning and maintenance of the apartment. When the landlord comes for the inspection, he is clearly surprised by the results and provides Stanley with positive feedback. ■ The occupational therapist creates cues for home maintenance. A cleaning schedule is created in which Stanley checks of the tasks he has finished at the end of the day. Stanley agrees that the most important concern is related to food being left out. A sign is placed at his door to the outside that reads "I will not leave the apartment until all dishes are clean and all food is stored properly." ■ The occupational therapist uses skills training approaches when addressing particular housekeeping tasks. For example, the occupational therapist instructs Stanley in vacuuming and explains how to start in one corner and systematically cover the whole floor. Practice with feedback is incorporated in the training. ■ The occupational therapist and Stanley identify options for helping Stanley stay motivated. Stanley decides that once per week he will invite a friend over to watch a movie or eat dinner together.

(continued)

Table 3. Case Descriptions: Adults With Serious Mental Illness *(cont.)*

Patient Description	Occupational Therapy Evaluation/Reevaluation	Occupational Therapy Goals	Occupational Therapy Interventions
Gerald, age 48, attends a consumer-operated program. During the last year he has gained a substantial amount of weight after an antipsychotic medication change related to symptoms associated with schizophrenia. He became more alarmed about his condition after a recent doctor's visit indicates Gerald has high blood pressure and symptoms of prediabetes.	▪ The initial weigh-in finds Gerald weighs 287 lbs. ▪ A 3-day food diary indicates that Gerald frequently eats out at fast food restaurants and chooses high-fat and high-calorie options from the bargain menu and that he drinks large amount of soda. ▪ Gerald reports that he does not engage in any regular physical activity but that in the past he enjoyed playing basketball. He lives close to the community college, which has an outdoor track.	▪ Gerald will lose at least 10 lbs during a 12-week weight-loss program. ▪ Gerald sets an initial goal of reducing his soda intake from 5 to 2 cans of soda a day. ▪ Gerald also plans to reduce the number of times that he eats at fast food restaurants to 3x/week and, when eating out, to make healthier selections. ▪ Gerald will engage in physical activity (walking or basketball) at least 4x/week for at least 30 minutes/session.	▪ Gerald attends a 12-week weight-loss program offered at the consumer operated program by an occupational therapist and co-led by a consumer provider. ▪ The weight loss program uses several strategies, including education and skills training related to nutrition and physical activity. ▪ During the group, the occupational therapist works more specifically with Gerald providing instruction on cooking simple, healthy meals at home and selecting healthier options at restaurants. ▪ During the group, the leaders recommend that group members get together outside the group for physical activity. Gerald and two other group members who live nearby make plans to play basketball together and walk on the track.

Note. IADLs = instrumental activities of daily living.

Table 4. Case Description: Occupational Therapist as Evaluator and Educator/Trainer

Patient Description	Referral to Occupational Therapy/ Occupational Therapy Evaluation	Occupational Therapy Goals Based on the OT Evaluation	Occupational Therapy Recommendations/Training
▪ **George, age 25,** lives in his own apartment in a supported living program with a job in a supportive workshop. He has a case manager and support staff to help with ADLs and IADLs. ▪ Reported diagnoses: bipolar disorder not otherwise specified, with psychotic features; learning disability (auditory processing disorder). ▪ Family history includes schizophrenia and bipolar disorder as well as a long history of problematic behaviors within the community. Because of his turbulent childhood, George has been difficult to place in group homes and apartment living. In his present	**Referral:** George was referred to occupational therapy by a government-administered community housing program to evaluate his current level of functioning in his daily routines; self-care and home management skills; and the resources necessary to support his physical and mental functioning, in particular within his present residential placement. **Evaluation:** ▪ Review of history ▪ Interviews with George and residential support staff ▪ Inventories (e.g., ADLs, interpersonal interactions, functional and social performance) completed by residential support staff	▪ Residential support staff (providers) will provide services in a way that matches George's functional requirements and increases his ability to access and utilize supports to maintain his community placement. ▪ Residential support staff will better understand George's functional requirements and related behaviors (that cause actions) to be able to work with him in a nonjudgmental manner. ▪ Residential support staff will demonstrate increased observation and communication skills with the following goals in mind: – To note and adapt approaches on the basis of George's functioning at the time of the interventions	**Program/system:** ▪ George should have access to 24-hour support for problem solving as issues occur. Support must be provided in a concrete, nonjudgmental manner within his level of information processing. **Environmental:** ▪ Residential support providers should give visual or gestured cues within George's immediate visual field, whenever teaching or providing cues for self-care and home management. ▪ All cueing and teaching of skills need to occur at the same time and follow the same patterns to support encoding of information into George's procedural memory.

(continued)

Table 4. Case Description: Occupational Therapist as Evaluator and Educator/Trainer *(cont.)*

Patient Description	Referral to Occupational Therapy/ Occupational Therapy Evaluation	Occupational Therapy Goals Based on the OT Evaluation	Occupational Therapy Recommendations/Training
supported living program, his interactions with his residential support staff are inconsistent, and his negative behaviors fluctuate, generally increasing after weekends with his family. He has a pattern of poor self-care and home management and exhibits stealing behaviors.	▪ Clinical observation in community interaction situations, work site, and home environments ▪ Standardized assessments (e.g., Allen's Cognitive Level Test and Routine Task Inventory; Adult Sensory Profile; Contextual Memory Test; Comprehensive Test of Visual Functioning	– To reduce negative interactions – To provide services as needed to support home management and self-care skills	▪ Tasks set up by residential support staff should be goal directed, concrete, and have strong manually manipulative properties in order to facilitate his ability to successfully complete them. ▪ George should be encouraged to include activities in his daily routine that involve comforting and organizing sensory inputs, as well as deep tactile and proprioceptive inputs to reduced behavioral incidents. **Training (Bathing routine):** ▪ Develop a plan for residential support staff to create a sensory comforting environment in George's bathing routine. ▪ Create a bathing routine that involves a consistent series of steps for George to follow to maintain the grooming skills required for his work environment.

Note. ADLs = activities of daily living; IADLs = instrumental activities of daily living. *Created by Linda T. Leonard, OTR/L.*

Summary of Evidence for Cognitive Interventions

Overall, the evidence examining cognitive interventions for people with serious mental illness is mixed. Although the evidence is inconsistent, there is greater support for cognitive remediation in terms of improving performance on specific cognitive tasks and less evidence for efficacy related to functional performance. For example, skills such as attention and memory improve with cognitive remediation, but this improvement does not appear to promote better community functioning; however, when the cognitive training is more closely linked to a real-world skill, the results are better.

Although the studies that have examined these constructs are few in number, cognitive adaptation training and errorless learning show promise for improving occupational performance in people with serious mental illness. In Tables 3 and 4 we list case studies that provide examples of evidence-based occupational therapy interventions.

Implications for Occupational Therapy Practice

This review has indicated there is significant evidence for many interventions within the domain of practice for occupational therapy that are effective in improving occupational performance. Occupational therapy practitioners must be "knowledgeable about evidence-based research and [apply] it ethically and appropriately to provide occupational therapy services consistent with best practice approaches" (AOTA, 2010, p. 417). The following general recommendations are based on the evidence

Table 5. Recommendations for Occupational Therapy Interventions for Adults With Serious Mental Illness

Areas of Occupation	Recommended	No Recommendation	Not Recom-mended
General	Supported employment or individual placement and support (IPS) programs to improve work placement in competitive employment and other vocational outcomes, in particular for those programs with high fidelity to the IPS model (A)	Supported employment programs to improve non-vocational outcomes (C)	Prevocational employment programs (D)
	Supported education programs to meet postsecondary education goals (B)	Ability to generalize life and social skills training from one environment or skill area to another (I)	
	Life and social skills training, with extended training in natural environments (B)		
	Skills training plus health care management (B)		
	Grocery shopping group to improve grocery shopping skills (C)		
	Parenting skills program (C)		
	Lifestyle interventions to improve health behaviors related to obesity and metabolic syndrome (A)		
	Physical activity, exercise, and outdoor activities improve symptoms of depression and anxiety (B)		
	Money management training (I)		
Performance Skills			
Cognitive	Cognitive remediation to improve life skills tied to real life practice (B)	Cognitive remediation to improve life skills without real-life practice (I)	
	Cognitive skills training in conjunction with supported employment (B)		
	Social cognition and problem-solving training (B)		
	Cognitive training to improve cognitive skills (B)		
Emotional regulation	Emotional regulation and social skills training in conjunction with supported employment (B)	Stress management in conjunction with a job program (I)	
	Activity group to improve social interaction skills (C)		
Performance Patterns			
Routines	Interpersonal and social rhythm therapy to establish and maintain routines for people with bipolar disorder (B)		
Roles	Client-centered role development program for the development of task and interpersonal skills within social roles (C)		
Context and environment	Environmental supports improve adaptive functioning (A)		
	Cooking skills are improved in both clinic and home environment (B)		
	In-home employment program to prepare for community-based employment (C)		
Activity demands	Use of a work behavior inventory to provide work-related feedback in combination with supported employment (B)		

Note. Recommendation criteria are based on the standard language of the Agency for Healthcare Research and Quality (2009). Suggested recommendations are based on the available evidence and content experts' opinions. ADL = activities of daily living.

A—Strongly recommend that occupational therapy practitioners routinely provide the intervention to eligible clients. Good evidence was found that the intervention improves important outcomes and concludes that benefits substantially outweigh harm.

B—Recommend that occupational therapy practitioners routinely provide the intervention to eligible clients. At least fair evidence was found that the intervention improves important outcomes and concludes that benefits outweigh harm.

C—There is weak evidence that the intervention can improve outcomes, and the balance of the benefits and harms may result either in a recommendation that occupational therapy practitioners routinely provide the intervention to eligible clients or in no recommendation because the balance of the benefits and harm is too close to justify a general recommendation.

D—Recommend that occupational therapy practitioners do not provide the intervention to eligible clients. At least fair evidence was found that the intervention is ineffective or that harm outweighs benefits.

I—Insufficient evidence to recommend for or against routinely providing the intervention. Evidence that the intervention is effective is lacking, of poor quality, or conflicting and the balance of benefits and harm cannot be determined.

described in this review (see Table 5 for more specific recommendations):

- Individuals with severe mental illness are able to acquire and maintain new knowledge and skills. Occupational therapy interventions should identify the specific knowledge and skills that are needed for an individual to succeed in the areas of occupation in which he or she needs or wants to succeed.
- Knowledge and skills-training outcomes are improved when the intervention is individualized, presented in a manner that is relevant and applicable to daily life, and incorporates training over an extended period of time (i.e., months as opposed to days or weeks).
- Client-centered practices that incorporate choice and collaboration promote better outcomes. Occupational therapists should seek input and create initial treatment plans that are based on the desires of the individual client.
- Improvements are most likely to occur in areas that are most proximal to the intervention; for example, cognitive interventions improve cognition, skills training results in improvements in the targeted skills, or supported employment most affects the client's ability to find a job. It is less likely that generalize ability of skills will occur without specific efforts toward that effect. For example, cognitive interventions generally do not result in occupational performance improvements unless they specifically target the occupation (e.g., cognitive-skills training incorporated in work or social-skills training). Occupational therapists, then, should select the intervention that most closely targets the desired outcome.
- Intervention in real-world environments is more effective than interventions that focus on pretraining or preliminary skill building; for example, the supported models (education and employment) indicate that pretraining is less effective than placement in actual work and educational settings and the training and support that are acquired in those real-world settings.

- Adapting the environment is a useful approach for improving occupational performance in individuals with serious mental illness. For example, cognitive adaptation training and job accommodations compensate for cognitive, sensory, and other impairments that interfere with successful community living. Occupational therapists are skilled in adapting the environment and can use this approach for addressing all areas of occupation.

Implications for Occupational Therapy Research

There is a growing body of occupational therapy research for people with serious mental illness, although occupational therapy has not played a primary role in the evidence base for this area of practice. Although there are many individual studies, there is a lack of cohesive evidence supporting interventions developed or implemented by occupational therapists. In this review, we have identified those interventions with the most established evidence base as those in which a manualized approach or some measure of fidelity to the intervention has been established.

Occupational therapists have been reluctant and/or slow to develop manualized interventions or fidelity measures. This may be due to an emphasis in the field of occupational therapy on individualization of service delivery that is consistent with recovery-oriented practice; however, intervention manuals do not negate individualization of services. Furthermore, manualization and fidelity scales promote the replication of intervention studies, make it easier to compare studies that propose to use the same intervention, and create greater transparency and understanding of a particular intervention approach. Occupational therapy researchers have a responsibility to society to develop intervention manuals or fidelity scales when designing interventions and intervention studies.

Implications for Occupational Therapy Education

In preparing occupational therapy practitioners to provide best practices, educators must keep abreast of the most current evidence. Occupational therapy education in mental health has not always focused on the most current evidence-based practices for people with serious mental illness. This practice guideline provides a valuable resource of current information that occupational therapy educators can use to develop the appropriate curricula. For example, occupational therapy educators should make sure that they are providing instruction that will prepare future therapists to provide evidence-based practices such as supported education, supported employment, skills training, and cognitive remediation. In addition, the evidence for practice is quickly evolving, and educators will need to identify additional strategies for augmenting these practice guidelines with the emergence of new evidence.

Appendix A.
Preparation and Qualifications of Occupational Therapists and Occupational Therapy Assistants

Who Are Occupational Therapists?

To practice as an occupational therapist, the individual trained in the United States

- Has graduated from an occupational therapy program accredited by the Accreditation Council for Occupational Therapy Education (ACOTE®) or predecessor organizations;
- Has successfully completed a period of supervised fieldwork experience required by the recognized educational institution where the applicant met the academic requirements of an educational program for occupational therapists that is accredited by ACOTE or predecessor organizations;
- Has passed a nationally recognized entry-level examination for occupational therapists; and
- Fulfills state requirements for licensure, certification, or registration.

Educational Programs for the Occupational Therapist

These include the following:

- Biological, physical, social, and behavioral sciences
- Basic tenets of occupational therapy
- Occupational therapy theoretical perspectives
- Screening evaluation
- Formulation and implementation of an intervention plan
- Context of service delivery
- Management of occupational therapy services (master's level)
- Leadership and management (doctoral level)
- Professional ethics, values, and responsibilities.

The fieldwork component of the program is designed to develop competent, entry-level, generalist occupational therapists by providing experience with a variety of clients across the life span and in a variety of settings. Fieldwork is integral to the program's curriculum design and includes an in-depth experience in delivering occupational therapy services to clients, focusing on the application of purposeful and meaningful occupation and/or research, administration, and management of occupational therapy services. The fieldwork experience is designed to promote clinical reasoning and reflective practice, to transmit the values and beliefs that enable ethical practice, and to develop professionalism and competence in career responsibilities. Doctoral-level students also must complete a doctoral experiential component designed to develop advanced skills beyond a generalist level.

Who Are Occupational Therapy Assistants?

To practice as an occupational therapy assistant, the individual trained in the United States

- Has graduated from an occupational therapy assistant program accredited by ACOTE or predecessor organizations;
- Has successfully completed a period of supervised fieldwork experience required by the recognized educational institution where the applicant met

the academic requirements of an educational program for occupational therapy assistants that is accredited by ACOTE or predecessor organizations;

- Has passed a nationally recognized entry-level examination for occupational therapy assistants; and
- Fulfills state requirements for licensure, certification, or registration.

Educational Programs for the Occupational Therapy Assistant

These include the following:
- Biological, physical, social, and behavioral sciences
- Basic tenets of occupational therapy
- Screening and assessment
- Intervention and implementation
- Context of service delivery
- Assistance in management of occupational therapy services
- Professional ethics, values, and responsibilities.

The fieldwork component of the program is designed to develop competent, entry-level, generalist occupational therapy assistants by providing experience with a variety of clients across the life span and in a variety of settings. Fieldwork is integral to the program's curriculum design and includes an in-depth experience in delivering occupational therapy services to clients, focusing on the application of purposeful and meaningful occupation. The fieldwork experience is designed to promote clinical reasoning appropriate to the occupational therapy assistant role, to transmit the values and beliefs that enable ethical practice, and to develop professionalism and competence in career responsibilities.

Regulation of Occupational Therapy Practice

All occupational therapists and occupational therapy assistants must practice under federal and state law. Currently, 50 states, the District of Columbia, Puerto Rico, and Guam have enacted laws regulating the practice of occupational therapy.

Note. The majority of this information is taken from the *Accreditation Standards for a Doctoral-Degree-Level Educational Program for the Occupational Therapist* (ACOTE, 2012a), *Accreditation Standards for a Master's-Degree-Level Educational Program for the Occupational Therapist* (ACOTE, 2012b), and *Accreditation Standards for an Educational Program for the Occupational Therapy Assistant* (ACOTE, 2012c).

Appendix B.
Evidence-Based Practice

One of the greatest challenges facing health care systems, service providers, public education, and policymakers is ensuring that scarce resources are used efficiently. The growing interest in outcomes research and evidence-based medicine over the past 30 years, and the more recent interest in evidence-based education, can in part be explained by these system-level challenges in the United States and internationally. In response to demands of the cost-oriented health care system in which occupational therapy practice is often embedded, occupational therapists and occupational therapy assistants are routinely asked to justify the value of the services they provide on the basis of the scientific evidence. The scientific literature provides an important source of legitimacy and authority for demonstrating the value of health care services. Thus, occupational therapy practitioners and other health care practitioners are increasingly called on to use the literature to demonstrate the value of the interventions and instruction they provide to clients.

According to Law and Baum (1998), *evidence-based occupational therapy practice* "uses research evidence together with clinical knowledge and reasoning to make decisions about interventions that are effective for a specific client" (p. 131). An evidence-based perspective is based on the assumption that scientific evidence of the effectiveness of occupational therapy intervention can be judged to be more or less strong and valid according to a hierarchy of research designs and an assessment of the quality of the research. The American Occupational Therapy Association (AOTA) uses standards of evidence modeled from those developed in evidence-based medicine. This model standardizes and ranks the value of scientific evidence for biomedical practice using the grading system in Table B1.

Level I, the highest level of evidence, includes studies that are systematic reviews of the literature, meta-analyses, and randomized controlled trials. In randomized controlled trials, the outcomes of an intervention are compared with the outcomes of a control group, and participation in either group is determined randomly. This design provides strength to the conclusion that the effect (dependent variable) was caused by the treatment (independent variable).

Level II evidence consists of studies in which assignment to a treatment or a control group is not randomized (i.e., a cohort study). *Level III* evidence consists of studies that do not use a control group. *Level IV* studies are experimental single-case studies, with at least marginal manipulation of the independent variable. *Level V* evidence includes descriptive case reports in which the authors present a description of the intervention/program and the outcome for the recipients of the service.

In this review, if Levels I, II, and III evidence for occupational therapy practice was adequate, then only those levels are used to answer a particular question. If, however, higher level evidence is lacking and the best evidence provided for occupational therapy specifically is ranked as only Levels IV and V, then studies at those levels are included.

Since 1998, AOTA has instituted a series of evidence-based practice (EBP) projects to assist its members in meeting the challenge of finding and reviewing the literature to identify evidence and,

Table B1. Levels of Evidence for Occupational Therapy Outcomes Research

Levels of Evidence	Definitions
Level I	Systematic reviews, meta-analyses, randomized controlled trials
Level II	Two groups, nonrandomized studies (e.g., cohort, case-control)
Level III	One group, nonrandomized (e.g., before and after, pretest and posttest)
Level IV	Descriptive studies that include analysis of outcomes (e.g., single-subject design, case series)
Level V	Case reports and expert opinion that include narrative literature reviews and consensus statements

Note. Adapted from "Evidence-Based Medicine: What It Is and What It Isn't," by D. L. Sackett, W. M. Rosenberg, J. A. Muir Gray, R. B. Haynes, & W. S. Richardson, 1996, *British Medical Journal, 312,* pp. 71–72. Copyright © 1996 by the British Medical Association. Adapted with permission.

in turn, using the findings from the evidence to inform practice (Lieberman & Scheer, 2002). Following the evidence-based philosophy of Sackett, Rosenberg, Gray, Haynes, and Richardson (1996), AOTA's projects are conducted based on the principle that the EBP of occupational therapy relies on the integration of information from three sources: (1) clinical experience and reasoning, (2) preferences of clients and their families, and (3) findings from the best available research.

A primary focus of AOTA's EBP projects is an ongoing program of systematic reviews of multidisciplinary scientific literature using focused questions and standardized procedures to identify practice-relevant evidence and discuss its implications for practice, education, and research. Systematic reviews of literature relevant to adults with serious mental illness strengthen our understanding of the foundations of this important area of practice.

Background

For many years, there have been ongoing efforts within AOTA to bring a stronger focus to the issue of mental health and occupational therapy. Part of these efforts included the appointment of several ad hoc groups to address the issues in mental health facing the profession that were integral to fulfilling AOTA's *Centennial Vision* (AOTA, 2007). The recommendations that resulted in a Representative Assembly motion in 2006 (Brown et al., 2006) were to create and disseminate evidence that supports occupational

therapy in mental health and to expand the evidence-based reviews to explore focused questions related to recovery-oriented outcomes in schizophrenia and mood disorders.

The evidence described herein presents the results of two systematic reviews developed through AOTA's Evidence-Based Literature Review Project. One systematic review was supported by AOTA as part of an academic partnership with Eastern Kentucky University (EKU) as a major investigation project fulfilling the master's-degree requirement for a nonthesis contribution. The second systematic review was supported by AOTA as part of an academic partnership with the Medical College of Georgia (MCG). Two occupational therapy students participated in the project in partial completion of the requirements for their master's degree.

Methodology

For the first academic partnership, three EKU graduate students, one faculty advisor, and AOTA project staff took part in the review. The EKU faculty advisor and AOTA staff developed the focused question. An advisory group consisting of occupational therapy practitioners, educators, and researchers with expertise in mental health provided input toward the development of the question. The EKU students, with support from AOTA staff and the advisory group, developed a search strategy to include the population, inclusion and exclusion criteria, and key search terms based on the population, interventions, and outcomes.

The key search terms for interventions were based on the following areas of occupation from the *Occupational Therapy Practice Framework: Domain and Process* (AOTA, 2008b): work, instrumental activities of daily living (including homemaking and cooking), and education. To operationalize serious mental illness, the group used the Center for Mental Health Services' definition requiring a person to have at least one 12-month disorder other than a substance use disorder, to meet criteria according to the *Diagnostic and Statistical Manual of Mental Disorders* (*DSM–IV–TR*; American Psychiatric Association, 2000), and to have serious impairment (Substance Abuse Mental Health Services Administration Public Health Services Act, 1993). Table B2 provides a comprehensive list of the search terms used for both systematic reviews.

Articles included in the review met the following criteria: published in a peer-reviewed journal, limited to English-language articles, participants had a diagnosis of severe mental illness and were between the ages of 18 and 65, and interventions were within the scope of occupational therapy practice. Only studies determined to be Level I (i.e., randomized controlled trials, systematic reviews, meta-analyses), Level II (i.e., nonrandomized clinical trials, cohort studies), and Level III (i.e., before–after, one-group designs) evidence were included. Studies were excluded if they were published before 1990, were Level IV or Level V evidence, used purely qualitative methods, were not peer reviewed, used geriatric or pediatric interventions, or used interventions outside the scope of occupational therapy practice. Databases searched included the Cumulative Index to Nursing and Allied Health Literature (CINAHL), MEDLINE, PsycINFO, HealthSTAR, Alternative Medicine (AMED), Social Work Abstracts, Cochrane Central Register of

Table B2. Search Terms for Systematic Review of Occupational Therapy Interventions for Adults With Serious Mental Illness

Categories	Key Search Terms
Patient/client population	Serious mental illness, chronic mental illness, serious and persistent mental illness, severe mental illness, personality disorder, anxiety disorder, psychosis, psychotic disorder, schizophrenia, mood disorder
Intervention	Child care (parenting, parents, child rearing, parent–child relations), meal preparation (menu planning, cooking, food-related skills, meal planning), home management (housekeeping, household management, laundry skills, ironing, repair, cleaning, gardening/yard work), shopping (grocery shopping, clothes shopping), time management (activity diary, individual time use, time, time factor, routines), safety (home safety, prevention, safety risks), education exploration (learning, career counseling, nonprofessional education), volunteer exploration (volunteerism, social participation, voluntary workers), retirement exploration (retiree), work exploration (occupation, vocation, job, employment, work), identifying an area of interest in work/education employment seeking (interest inventories, interests, personality traits, vocational interests, self-evaluation, career planning, vocational aptitude), employment seeking (interviewing, vocational rehabilitation, resume writing, employability, job search, assistance, sheltered workshops, employment, unemployment), job performance (work performance, employee attitude, work ethic, schedules, work tolerance, occupational stress, work environment, work habits, routines, relationships, compliance with rules/policies)
	Communication interaction in relation to employment, volunteer, home management, child care (interpersonal relations, verbal/nonverbal processing abilities, communication counseling, listening skills, conversational skills, social communication, communicative skills); simulated/practice in employment, volunteer, home management, child care (psychodrama, social stories, simulation, modeling, coaching); decision making (decision making skills, problem solving, problem-solving skills, thinking skills); activity groups in volunteer, home management, child care (programming, group counseling, group work, occupational therapy groups); skill training (living skills training, social skills training, community living skills training, self management, functional adaptation skills training, psychosocial intervention, everyday living skills training, daily living skills); psychosocial clubs (Fountain House, clubhouse); assertive community treatment; psychosocial rehabilitation; psychiatric rehabilitation
Comparison	N/A
Outcomes	Occupational performance and role competence in paid and unpaid employment (volunteer opportunities, home management, education)

Controlled Trials and Database of Systemic Reviews, Database of Abstracts of Effects, American College of Physicians (ACP) Journal Club, and OT Seeker.

An initial search was completed in conjunction with a research librarian at EKU. In addition, a medical librarian with experience in conducting systematic reviews completed a second search using a filter based on one developed at McMaster University (http://www.urmc.rochester.edu/hslt/miner/digital_library/evidence_based_resources.cfm). The list of 950 citations and abstracts from both searches was reviewed, and 145 potential articles were evaluated according to inclusion and exclusion criteria. Articles selected for inclusion were analyzed and critically appraised, and individual articles were summarized in an evidence table. A Critically Appraised Topic (CAT) further summarized and synthesized the information, and both the evidence table and CAT were submitted to AOTA staff and the project consultant for review. The students presented on the review process and the AOTA collaboration as a component of requirements for their master's project. A total of 46 articles were selected for final analysis in the review. Of those, 37 were Level I studies, 5 were Level II studies, and 4 were Level III studies.

For the academic partnership with MCG, an advisory group consisting of occupational therapy practitioners, educators (including MCG faculty) and researchers with expertise in mental health, AOTA staff, and a consultant to AOTA's EBP projects developed the focused question for the systematic review. The MCG team, with support from AOTA staff and the advisory group, developed a search strategy to include the population; inclusion and exclusion criteria; and key search terms based on the population, interventions, and outcomes using the same search terms developed by the EKU group. Articles included in the review met the following criteria: published in a peer-reviewed journal, limited to English language, participants had a diagnosis of severe mental illness and were between the ages of 18 and 65, and interventions were within the scope of occupational therapy practice.

Only studies determined to be Level I, Level II, or Level III evidence were included. Studies were excluded if they were published before 1990, were Level IV or V evidence, used purely qualitative methods, were not peer reviewed, were limited to geriatric or pediatric populations, or used interventions outside the scope of occupational therapy practice. Databases searched included CINAHL, MEDLINE, PsycINFO, HealthSTAR, AMED, Social Work Abstracts, Cochrane Central Register of Controlled Trials and Database of Systemic Reviews, Database of Abstracts of Effects, ACP Journal Club, and OT Seeker.

The search of the databases was completed by a medical librarian with experience in conducting systematic reviews using a filter based on one developed at McMaster University (http://www.urmc.rochester.edu/hslt/miner/digital_ library/evidence_based_resources.cfm). Abstracts were sought for all citations from this review. All abstracts were downloaded into Zotero (http://www.zotero.org), a free Web-based citation manager extension of Mozilla Firefox that was used to manage all abstracts and articles.

All 1,964 abstracts identified by the search process were reviewed by at least three individuals working on the project using the inclusion/exclusion criteria described above. A total of 101 articles were acquired and assigned to individual reviewers. After further review, some of the articles were found to not meet the inclusion criteria and were excluded from the final review. Additional articles were identified from reviews of reference lists and hand searches. The remaining 50 articles that met all inclusion criteria were analyzed and critically appraised and summarized in an evidence table. A CAT further summarized and synthesized the information, and both the evidence table and CAT were submitted to AOTA staff and the project consultant for review.

The findings from studies included in the systematic reviews also were used to develop evidence-based recommendations. These recommendations for occupational therapy practice for adults with serious mental illness can be found in Table 5 of the main document. The recommendations are based on the strength of the evidence for a given topic from the systematic reviews in combination with the expert opinions of the review authors and content experts reviewing this guideline. The strength of the evidence is determined by the number of articles included in a given topic, the study design, and limitations of those articles. The review authors and other content experts provided clinical expertise regarding the value of using a given intervention in practice. Recommendation criteria are based on standard language developed by the U.S. Preventive Services Task Force of the Agency for Health Care Research and Quality. More information regarding these criteria can be found at http://www.uspreventiveservicestaskforce.org/uspstf/standard.htm.

Thirty-one of the articles included in the review were Level I studies, 13 were Level II studies, and 6 were Level III studies. The evidence table of all articles included in both reviews can be found in Appendix C. A total of 96 articles were included in the review of the two focused questions. Although the review included published literature from occupational therapy as well as related fields, all studies provided evidence within the scope of occupational therapy practice. Sixty-seven (71%) of the articles were at Level I, and 85 (89%) of the articles were at Level I or Level II, indicating that the review incorporated evidence at the highest levels.

Limitations in several of the studies incorporated into the review included lack of randomization, lack of a control group, small sample size, lack of blinding of researcher to treatment allocation, limited follow-up, and sampling bias. In several studies, the dropout rate by participants was large and may not have been documented. In addition, several studies did not describe the experimental and control conditions, and in others, the intervention and comparison groups varied with respect to intensity of intervention. In some studies, the validity of the outcome measure was not reported, and in several, the outcome measures were similar to the intervention. The definition or description of occupational therapy programs also varied from study to study. Generalization of results of a number of studies was limited when a study was gender-specific or the study did not take place in the United States.

Appendix C.
Evidence Tables

Evidence Table 1. Mental Health Recovery Model in the Areas of Community Integration and Normative Life Roles

Author/Year	Study Objectives	Level/Design/Participants	Intervention and Outcome Measures	Results	Study Limitations
Level I					
Anzai et al. (2002)	Examine effectiveness of the Community Re-entry Model when adapted for Japanese psychiatric patients in teaching the knowledge and skills required to live and participate in the community	I—Randomized controlled trial $N = 29$ Group 1 = 14 Group 2 = 15 Mean duration of illness: 20.5 years Mean age: 46.8 years Mean hospitalization: 4 years	*Intervention:* Group 1: Community Re-entry Module: highly structured curriculum that consists of sessions on medication, relapse, finding housing and psychiatric care in the community, reducing stress, and coping Group 2 (control): Conventional occupational rehabilitation program, consisting of arts and crafts, reality orientation groups, and work assignments in the hospital *Outcome Measures:* ■ Hospital discharge rates; ■ REHAB Scale ■ A 21-item instrument from Community Re-entry module	Group 1 had significant increase in knowledge and skills on a 21-item instrument at 1-year follow-up. Group 2 showed no significant gains. 10 of 14 Group 1 members were discharged from the hospital; only 3 from Group 2 were discharged. At 1-year follow-ups, the Community Re-entry group lost some skills but were still significantly higher than baseline. On the REHAB scale, Group 1 had improved scores and Group 2 had no change.	Small group sizes. Conducted in Japan. Focus of measurement was medication management that was specifically taught to one group but not the other.
Beynon, Soares-Weiser, Woolacott, Duffy, & Geddes (2008)	Determine the effectiveness of psychosocial intervention for the prevention of relapse in bipolar disorder	I—Systematic review and meta-analysis $N = 12$ studies involving psychosocial interventions of a adults with bipolar disorder I or II	*Intervention:* Interventions included cognitive–behavioral therapy (CBT), family therapy, group psycho-education, case management, and integrated group therapy. *Outcome Measures:* Defined as relapse that required rehospitalization or the need for additional treatment	CBT in combination with usual treatment is effective in preventing relapse. There is reasonably good evidence that group psycho-education is more effective than nonstructured groups in preventing relapse. Family therapy was found not to be more effective in reducing relapse; however, the comparison groups involved used active therapy, which could have reduced differences in outcomes. Insufficient evidence exists to fully evaluate care management and integrated group therapy.	In general, studies that investigated psychosocial interventions were small, and there was varied quality. There was an insufficient number of studies to determine whether one approach was better than the others in reducing relapse.

(continued)

Evidence Table 1. Mental Health Recovery Model in the Areas of Community Integration and Normative Life Roles *(continued)*

Author/Year	Study Objectives	Level/Design/Participants	Intervention and Outcome Measures	Results	Study Limitations
Buchain, Vizzotto, Henna Neto, & Elkis (2002)	Determine the effectiveness of occupational therapy in conjunction with pharmaceutical interventions on social skills in clients with treatment-resistant schizophrenia	I—Randomized controlled trial $N = 26$ Experimental group, $n = 14$ Control group, $n = 12$	*Intervention:* The experimental group received a combination of occupational therapy and clozapine. Participants had a free choice of activities performed within the group. The control group received only clozapine. *Outcome Measures:* Participants were assessed at baseline and monthly, or a total of 7 times with the Scale of Interactive Observation in Occupational Therapy.	Occupational therapy intervention was more effective overall with appropriate medication than medication alone, particularly from Month 4 to the end of the study.	The means by which the authors determined the statistical findings was not clear. Small sample size and large attrition. The study was conducted in Brazil; thus the results may not generalize to U.S. samples.
Cabassa, Ezell, & Lewis-Fernandez (2010)	Evaluate the effectiveness of lifestyle intervention outcome studies to lower risk and morbidity associated with obesity, cardiovascular disease, and diabetes for persons with serious mental illness	I—Systematic review $N = 23$ studies: randomized and nonrandomized controlled trial, and single-group studies, published between 1980 and 2009	*Intervention:* Lifestyle interventions provided to persons with serious mental illness included weight management, cognitive–behavioral treatment, physical activity, and exercise. *Outcome Measures:* Outcomes included weight, BMI, blood pressure, and health promotion (e.g., self-efficacy, health-related quality of life).	12 of 23 studies reported significant improvements either in weight loss or metabolic syndrome risk factors in participants who took part in a lifestyle intervention program.	Limitations of the studies incorporated into the review include numerous outcome measures, small sample sizes, and heterogeneity of study designs.
Chafetz, White, Collins-Bride, Cooper, & Nickens (2008)	Evaluate the effectiveness of the addition of a wellness training (WT) program to standard care (basic primary care; BPC) for individuals with significant mental illness to improve perceived health status, self-efficacy, and psychosocial function	I—Randomized controlled trial $N = 309$ BPC, $n = 154$ WT, $n = 155$ Participants were recruited from short-term crisis residential units. Diagnostic conditions primarily included depressive disorders, schizophrenia, and bipolar affective disorders. Exclusion criteria included dementia or a single diagnosis of an adjustment disorder.	*Intervention:* Usual care (BPC) is an established part of a crisis residential unit (health assessments, immediate or short-term care, health education, and referrals). Intervention included up to 12 months of WT (an individually administered, manualized skills training program, The Personal Health Profile). Clients were interviewed at baseline, 6 months, 12 months, and 18 months. *Outcome Measures:* ■ Medical Outcomes Health Survey Short Form 36 (SF–36) ■ Health-related self-efficacy ■ Global Assessment of Functioning (GAF) to assess psychosocial function	Significant differences in linear change by study group were found on the SF–36 Physical Functioning and General Health scales, controlling for baseline severity of illness and the alcohol and drug scores measured at each interview. Other scales of the SF–36 did not differ by study group; neither did scores for self-efficacy or the GAF.	Higher attrition in the WT group during follow-up interviews. Reliance on self-reported data. Small number of WT participants actively used the services available.

Author/Year	Study Objectives	Level/Design	Intervention and Outcome Measures	Results	Study Limitations
Chan, Lee, & Chan (2007)	Compare the Transforming Relapse and Instilling Prosperity (TRIP) ward program led by occupational therapists with traditional activities-based ward occupational therapy (WOT) in an acute care setting	I—Randomized controlled trial

$N = 81$
TRIP, $n = 44$
WOT, $n = 37$

18- to 63-year-old males; diagnosis of schizophrenia or schizoaffective disorder | *Intervention:*
TRIP consisted of 10 sessions related to illness management and health promotion conducted by an occupational therapist using a semi-structured format with didactic presentation followed by open discussion.

WOT had an equivalent length of time and frequency as TRIP. It consisted of a normal routine selected by the clients. Content included clerical or craft work tasks and recreational and leisure activities.

Outcome Measures:
- Scale of Unawareness of Mental Disorder (SUMD)
- SF–36 Medical Outcomes scale
Readmission rates were counted at 3 months to 12 months, with odds ratio relapse rates calculated. | Sociodemographically, the groups were comparable; a pre- and posttest SUMD and SF–36 between-groups analysis of covariance revealed significant improvement for TRIP group members in the physical health component and mental health component and their perceived health. Relapse rates were lower for the TRIP group between the 9- and 12-month follow-up period as compared with the WOT group, with a 1.75 odds ratio for the WOT group members indicating that they were almost 2× more likely to be rehospitalized within 12 months. | Study only included males and took place in Hong Kong, so the results may not generalize to the U.S. population. |
| Choi & Kwon (2006) | Evaluate whether Social Cognition Enhancement Training (SCET) improves social cognitive abilities for individuals with schizophrenia and examine the pattern of changes in the three phases of training | I—Randomized controlled trial

$N = 34$ (19 men, 15 women) from community-based psychiatric rehabilitation centers in Korea

Participants had a diagnosis of schizophrenia or schizoaffective disorder, were ages 18–60, and were taking stabilizing antipsychotic medications. | *Intervention:*
SCET plus standard psychiatric rehabilitation training compared with just standard psych rehabilitation training. SCET included a package of 36 sessions, 2×/wk for 6 months in a group setting; it included social cognitive exercises, discussion, and problem solving.

Standard treatment included a comprehensive program to improve daily coping skills, optimize medication adherence, and increase social and occupational functioning.

The treatment team included a social worker, psychologist, nurse, and/or occupational therapist who acted as case manager and provided discipline-specific treatment guided by psychosocial rehabilitation principles.

Outcome Measures:
- Picture Arrangement (PA) section of Wechsler Intelligence Scale for Children–Revised
- Social Behavioral Sequencing Task (SBCT)
- Contextual Recognition of the Emotional Recognition Test (CR–ERT) | Phase effects of SCET: PA scores exhibited significant differences between groups at the 4-month and 6-month posttreatment follow-up (Phases 2 and 3, respectively). SBCT showed significant differences between groups at the 2-month measurement (Phase 1); no significant difference were shown between groups on the CR–ERT. | Approximately 50% of participants did not complete the study.
Small sample size.
Length of intervention may cause increase in dropout rate.
Unable to determine whether understanding of social situations transfers to improved interpersonal transactions.
Limited generalize ability. |

(continued)

Evidence Table 1. Mental Health Recovery Model in the Areas of Community Integration and Normative Life Roles (continued)

Author/Year	Study Objectives	Level/Design/Participants	Intervention and Outcome Measures	Results	Study Limitations
Cook, Chambers, & Coleman (2009)	Investigate the effectiveness of occupational therapy for people with psychotic conditions	I—Pilot randomized controlled trial with stratified randomization by gender and treatment team Assessors were blinded to the intervention. $N = 44$ adults with psychosis and other psychotic conditions over age 16. Occupational therapy, $n = 30$ Treatment as usual (TAU; control), $n = 14$	*Intervention:* Occupational therapy: Up to 12 months of individual occupational therapy in community settings as an adjunct to standard care. The intervention schedule was defined and not highly structured so as to reflect standard occupational therapy practice. The TAU condition was delivered by non-occupational therapy staff and involved medications, care coordination, and supportive interventions for 12 months. *Outcome Measures:* Assessed at baseline and then at 6, 12, and 18 months. • Social Functioning Scale • Scale for the Assessment of Negative Symptoms • Employment	Both groups demonstrated improvement; however, there was no difference between groups on the outcomes measures. The members of the occupational therapy group showed clinically significant improvements not apparent in the TAU group on four subscales of the Social Functioning Scale: Relationships, Independence Performance, Independence Competence, and Recreation.	Some members of the control group received occupational therapy. Power and effect size were not determined prior to study; therefore, the study may have had insufficient numbers to demonstrate a treatment effect difference. Measurement did not appear to capture the effect of occupational therapy.
Dilk & Bond (1996)	Analyze the effectiveness of skills training for individuals with severe mental illness	I—Meta-analysis $N = 68$ articles published between 1970 and 1992, doctoral dissertations, and master's theses Studies with at least 5 participants, Levels I, II, and III	*Intervention:* Training programs taught the following skills: general interpersonal, assertiveness, prevocational, assertiveness, micro-interpersonal, dating, affective management, cognitive. Training approaches were either behavioral or cognitive–behavioral. Settings included both inpatient and outpatient. *Outcome Measures:* • Skill acquisition • Symptom reduction • Personal adjustment • Hospitalization • Vocational readiness	Skills training was found to be moderately to strongly effective in teaching inpatients interpersonal and assertiveness skills and reducing psychiatric symptoms. Effect sizes varied by outcome measures, with context-specific measures resulting in larger outcomes than skill usage and role functioning.	Research studies rarely evaluated use of trained skills. Limited number of studies examining skills training in settings other than psychiatric hospitals. Because many of the outcome measures were similar to the studied interventions, the authors warn against the generalize ability of the results. Gender and ethnicity was not evenly represented

Author/Year	Study Objectives	Level/Design/Participants	Intervention and Outcome Measures	Results	Study Limitations
Duncombe (2004)	Determine whether there is a difference between learning the functional living skill of cooking for people with serious and persistent schizophrenia when it is taught in a clinic or in their home	I—Randomized controlled trial $N = 44$ participants with a diagnosis of nonparanoid schizophrenia or schizoaffective living in group homes or supported apartments that had kitchens available. Participants were assigned in 22 pairs matched on cognitive level and randomly assigned to 1 of 2 groups.	*Intervention:* Group 1: Cooking skills training in the home Group 2: Cooking skills training in the clinic. Participants received treatment individually 4 times in the designated context with a 1-wk lapse between each session. *Outcome Measures:* Kitchen Task Assessment–Modified (KTA–M)	Both groups posted significant improvement between their pre- and post-treatment scores on the KTA–M. The results did not show a significant difference in the level of learning between the 2 groups in the different contexts.	Qualitative differences in the 2 settings may have affected the results. The clinic was quiet with minimal distractions. The kitchens in the group homes were cluttered and distracting. Multiple intervention sites result in inconsistencies in the research. There may have been a ceiling effect for the KTA–M.
Dunn, Trivedi, Kampert, Clark, & Chambliss (2005)	Evaluate the effectiveness of exercise for the treatment of mild to moderate major depressive disorder (MDD)	I—Randomized controlled trial $N = 80$ adults with MDD $n = 16$, low-dose (LD), $3\times/wk$ $N = 18$, LD, $5\times/wk$ $n = 17$ public health dose (PHD), $3\times/wk$ $n = 16$, PHD, $5\times/wk$ $n = 13$, control (stretching, $3\times/wk$)	*Intervention:* Participants were randomized to the LD or higher PHD condition or the control group. Exercises took place in a supervised laboratory setting. *Outcome Measures:* ■ Hamilton Rating Scale for Depression $(HRSD_{17})$ ■ Response rate ■ Remission rate	There was a significant effect on $HRSD_{17}$ scores at 12 wk. The scores were reduced 47% for the PHD group, 30% for the LD group, and 29% for the control group. Participants in the PHD condition were significantly less likely to have a remission as compared with those in the control condition. There was no difference in remission between the PHD and LD groups.	Due to lack of blinding to treatment condition, there was a high dropout rate for the control group. There was a relatively small sample per group. Authors reported that the use of a laboratory setting may reduce the ability to generalize the results to clinical practice.
Dunn, Trivedi, & O'Neal (2001)	Examine scientific evidence for a dose–response relation of physical activity with depressive and anxiety disorders	I—Systematic review $N = 37$ articles Study participants had depression or anxiety as the primary disorder.	9 cross-sectional and 9 prospective studies addressed dose–response effects of total amount of leisure time and occupational physical activity; 19 studies addressed exercise training studies, including aerobic and resistance training protocols.	An association was found between increased activity and decreased depression. Exercise training studies: 8 studies reported a 50% reduction in anxiety/depression. Both resistance and aerobic exercise were effective in reducing symptoms of depression.	Most studies addressed depression, not anxiety. Few addressed the dose–response relationship.

(continued)

Evidence Table 1. Mental Health Recovery Model in the Areas of Community Integration and Normative Life Roles *(continued)*

Author/Year	Study Objectives	Level/Design/Participants	Intervention and Outcome Measures	Results	Study Limitations
Edgelow & Krupa (2011)	Evaluate the effectiveness of Action Over Inertia, an occupational time-use intervention to improve occupational balance and engagement among community-dwelling individuals with serious mental illness	I—Randomized controlled trial *N* = 24 community-dwelling people with serious mental illness receiving assertive community treatment services At completion of study, *n* = 8 control (standard care) participants and *n* = 10 treatment participants	*Intervention* Action Over Inertia, a workbook format that individualizes increasing occupational activity to promote health and well-being and focuses on managing change and goal-planning. *Outcome Measures:* ■ 24-hr time diaries ■ Profiles of Occupational Engagement for People with Schizophrenia ■ Feedback of clinical utility	Participants in the Action Over Inertia group increased their occupational balance by spending an average of 47 min more per day in activity than the control group (*p* = .05). Although there were no differences between groups for occupational engagement, the authors reported evidence of clinical utility.	Small sample size; lack of follow-up data; treatment group was older and had a longer time to diagnosis than the control group.
Frank et al. (2005)	Compare interpersonal and social rhythm therapy (IPSRT) and intensive clinical management (ICM) in the treatment of bipolar I disorder	I—Randomized controlled trial *N* = 175 participants with a lifetime history of bipolar Type I disorder or schizoaffective disorder, manic type *n* = 43, ICM/ICM acute/maintenance phase *n* = 45, ICM/IPSRT *n* = 48, IPSRT/ICM *n* = 39, IPSRT/IPSRT	*Intervention:* Participants were randomized to groups based on ICM or IPSRT in the acute phase, followed by ICM or IPSRT in the maintenance phase. IPSRT stresses the importance of maintaining daily routines and identifying potential rhythm disruptors. ICM is a manual-driven approach to the medical management of bipolar disorder that includes education about the disorder, medications, and sleep hygiene, and nonspecific support. *Outcome Measures:* ■ Time to stabilization in the acute phase and time to recurrence in the maintenance phase ■ Social Rhythm Metric	There was no difference between groups for time to stabilization. Participants in IPSRT in the acute phase survived longer without a new episode regardless of treatment approach in the maintenance phase. In addition, those in IPSRT had higher regularity of social rhythms at the end of acute treatment.	Variables that were later found to be associated with outcome, such as marital status and medical burden, were not distributed equally among the maintenance study conditions.

56

Adults With Serious Mental Illness

Author/Year	Study Objectives	Level/Design/Participants	Intervention and Outcome Measures	Results	Limitations/Comments
Glynn et al. (2002)	Compare the effectiveness of clinic-based skills training vs. skills training augmented with formal practice within the community to demonstrate generalize ability	I—Randomized controlled trial *N* = 63 participants between ages of 18 and 60 with a *DSM–IV* diagnosis of schizophrenia or schizophrenia disorder. Group 1: *n* = 32 Group 2: *n* = 31	*Intervention:* Group 1: Treatment with Risperidone or Haloperidol and behaviorally oriented clinic-based social skills training either alone or Group 2: In conjunction with in vivo amplified skills training). *Outcome Measures:* Module tests at baseline and at 24 wk ■ Patient version of the Social Adjustment Scale–II ■ Quality of Life Scale ■ The Social Adjustment Scale–II was administered at baseline, 36 wk, and 60 wk. The Quality of Life Scale was administered at baseline and then every 12 wk through Week 60.	Participation in clinic-based plus in-vivo amplified skills training was associated with significantly greater improvements in instrumental role functioning and overall adjustment as assessed with the Social Adjustment Scale–II. Both conditions showed improvements on the Quality of Life Scale instrumental role, intrapsychic motivation, common objects, and overall composite scores. Participants who participated in clinic-based plus in vivo amplified skills training improved more quickly, and often to higher levels, than the clinic-based skills training alone.	28% loss of participants over 60 wk without clear explanation of intent-to-treat analyses. 2 intervention groups varied in intensity of their treatment; in vivo amplified skills training received more contact with mental health professionals.
Granholm et al. (2005)	Compare usual treatment vs. usual treatment plus cognitive–behavioral social skills training on social functioning, psychotic and depressive symptoms, cognitive insight, and skill mastery	I—Randomized controlled trial *N* = 76 community-dwelling adults diagnosed with schizophrenia or schizoaffective Age: 42–74 years old. *n* = 37 cognitive–behavioral group *n* = 39 control group	*Intervention:* Cognitive–behavioral social skills training group received 24 weekly, 2-hr group psycho-therapy sessions including homework forms/workbooks, received training modules. Control group: Treatment as usual. *Outcome Measures:* ■ Cognitive Therapy Rating Scale for Psychosis ■ Independent Living Skills Survey and USCD Positive and Negative Syndrome Scale and Hamilton Rating Scale ■ Beck Cognitive Insight Scale ■ Comprehensive Module Test	At end of 6 months, participants in the cognitive–behavioral social group performed social functioning activities more frequently than other group; however, they showed no significant improvement when performing everyday functional activities after treatment. Group receiving usual treatment alone showed increased score on the Hamilton depression scale at the 3rd month assessment. No report of any benefit linked to the repetition of the cognitive behavioral modules.	Authors report a moderately small sample size, and exclusion of patients with comorbid conditions may limit generalize ability.

(continued)

Evidence Table 1. Mental Health Recovery Model in the Areas of Community Integration and Normative Life Roles (continued)

Author/Year	Study Objectives	Level/Design/Participants	Intervention and Outcome Measures	Results	Study Limitations
Grawe, Falloon, Widen, & Skogvoll (2006)	Evaluate the benefits derived from continued integrated biomedical and psychosocial intervention for recent-onset schizophrenia	I—Randomized controlled study N = 50 individuals with schizophrenia n = 30 Integrated treatment (IT) n = 20 Standard treatment (ST)	*Intervention:* ST: Patients received regular clinic-based case management with antipsychotic drugs, supportive housing and day care, crisis inpatient treatment, rehabilitation that promoted independent living and work activity, brief psycho-education, and supportive psychotherapy. IT: Patients treated by multidisciplinary team independent of the ST program. In addition to ST, IT cases received structured family psychoeducation, cognitive–behavioral family communication and problem-solving skills training, intensive crisis management provided at home, and individual cognitive–behavioral strategies for residual symptoms and disability. *Outcome Measures:* ▪ Target Psychiatric Symptoms ▪ Composite Clinical Index ▪ Brief Psychiatric Rating Scale ▪ Global Assessment of Functioning	IT group was superior to ST in reducing negative symptoms, minor psychotic episodes, and in stabilizing positive symptoms, but did not reduce hospital admissions or major psychotic recurrences. More IT patients had better 2-year outcomes than ST patients.	Moderately small sample size.
Kopelowicz, Wallace, & Zarate (1998)	Examine the effects of a brief manualized treatment program of skills to reenter the community and actively follow through with their own care	I—Randomized controlled trial N = 59 adults with a diagnosis of schizophrenia or schizoaffective disorder Community reentry, n = 28, Occupational therapy, n = 31	*Intervention:* Community reentry treatment was based on the Social and Independent Living Skills Modules developed at the UCLA, and modified for use in the rapid turnover, "crisis" operations of a typical acute psychiatric inpatient facility. It consists of 16 training sessions of 45 min divided into 2 8-session sections and includes skills needed to avoid illicit drugs, cope with stress, organize a daily schedule, and make and keep appointments with service providers. Occupational therapy included a full range of customary occupational therapy activities conducted by 2–3 occupational therapists. *Outcome Measures:* ▪ Test of Knowledge and Performance (18 questions, problems and role plays, and interviews [which were videotaped] related to session info) ▪ Attendance at after services	Test scores following intervention were 81% correct for reentry program vs. 55% for the occupational therapy program. Clients in the reentry program were significantly more likely to keep postdischarge appointments than were occupational therapy participants.	Limited population, description of occupational therapy, and outcome measures.

Author/Year	Study Objectives	Level/Design/Sample	Intervention and Outcome Measures	Results	Limitations
Kopelowicz, Zarate, Smith, Mintz, & Liberman (2003)	Evaluate the effectiveness of skills training program designed to teach disease management to Latinos with schizophrenia treated in a community mental health center	I—Randomized controlled trial N = 92 Latinos outpatients 18–60 years old, and family members Skills Training Group, n = 45 members, 39 completed Customary Outpatient Care n = 47 members, 45 completed	*Intervention:* 3 months of skills training or customary care, then followed for a total of 9 months. Program was culturally adapted through input of patient's key relatives. *Outcome Measures:* <ul><li>Positive and negative Syndrome Scale</li><li>Los Angeles County Dept Mental Health Management Information System</li><li>Independent Living Skills Survey</li><li>Quality of Life Interview</li><li>Rating of Medication Influences Scale</li><li>Interview and Role Playing based on Skills Modules</li></ul>Outcome measures for family participants: Patient's Future Scale, Miller Hope Scale, Five Minute Speech Sample, Camberwell Family Interview, Family Burden Interview Schedule	The results indicate that those in the skills training group had more skills acquisition and generalization that those in the control group. There was no statistically significant difference between groups for quality of life, caregiver burden, adherence to medication, and attitude toward medication. Rehospitalization and family measures had no statistical significance between groups; however, more people were re-hospitalized in the control group at 9- and 15-month reports	Relatively limited follow-up.
Kurtz, Seltzer, Shagan, Thime, & Wexler (2007)	Evaluate the effects of a treatment with computer-assisted cognitive remediation that included explicit training in attention verbal and nonverbal working and episodic memory, and language processing exercises	I—Randomized controlled trial, single blind N = 42 outpatients with schizophrenia or schizoaffective disorder participated. Cognitive remediation, n = 23 Computer training, n = 19	*Intervention:* 12-month standardized course of cognitive remediation consisting of a sequence of computerized cognitive exercises designed to improve attention, verbal and nonverbal memory, and language processing through repeated drill and practice. Control: Similar exposure to computer and clinician, with non-specific cognitive challenge. *Outcome Measures:* <ul><li>Working memory: The Digit Span, Arithmetic and Letter–Number sequencing subtests from the WAIS–III; Verbal Episodic memory</li><li>Logical memory; Speed of information processing: the Digit Symbol and Symbol Search subtests from the WAIS–III, Trailmaking test, Grooved Pegboard and Letter Fluency</li><li>Visual episodic memory: Rey Complex Figure Test; Reasoning; Penn Conditional Exclusion Test, and Booklet Category Test</li></ul>	Cognitive remediation yields significant improvement in working memory. Other domains show similar progress across both groups. No significant differences were evident between cognitive remediation or computer skills training groups for demographic, clinical, or treatment variables. ANOVA for each of the 5 neuro-cognitive domains revealed main effects of time for working memory, verbal episodic, memory, spatial episodic memory, processing speed and reasoning/executive function suggesting participants in both groups improved.	Small sample size; relationships among some variables remains unclear; study did not include an independent measure of cognitive challenge based on performance of functional activity.

(continued)

Evidence Table 1. Mental Health Recovery Model in the Areas of Community Integration and Normative Life Roles (*continued*)

Author/Year	Study Objectives	Level/Design/Participants	Intervention and Outcome Measures	Results	Study Limitations
Liberman et al. (1998)	Compare community functioning of outpatients with severe and persistent form of schizophrenia following treatment with occupational therapy or skills training	I—Randomized, controlled trial, blinded *N* = 84 men living in the community with persistent forms of schizophrenia Mean age: 37.1 years	*Intervention:* 6 months of intensive clinic-based treatment in 1 of 2 groups. Skills training: Modules taught by an occupational therapist and paraprofessionals included basic conversation, recreation for leisure, medication management, and symptom management. Psychosocial occupational therapy: Expressive, artistic, and recreational activities. *Outcome Measures:* ■ Independent Living Skills Survey ■ Social Activities Scale, Profile of Adaptation to Life	The cohort receiving the social skills training achieved significantly higher total scores on the Independent Living Skills assessment. Differences were most marked at 6 months but diminished and were not significant at 12 and 24 months.	Limited accounting of attrition in results.
Lindenmayer et al. (2008)	Evaluate the feasibility and efficacy of a cognitive remediation program to improve cognitive and work functioning	I—Randomized controlled trial *N* = 85 (89% male) Cognitive remediation, *n* = 45, Control group, *n* = 40 Participants were intermediate- to long-term inpatients at a psychiatric treatment center. Diagnoses included schizophrenia and bipolar disorder.	*Intervention:* Intervention was a 12-wk computerized cognitive remediation program that consisted of 2 hr computer time and 1 hr group discussion application time. Control members participated in 3 hr game or instructional time on the computer per week. All participants took part in mandatory unit activities up to 20 hr/wk. *Outcome Measures:* ■ Cognitive functioning, including attention, psychomotor speed, verbal working memory, and executive function ■ Work activity ■ Positive and Negative Symptom Scale (PANSS)	Participants in the cognitive training group demonstrated significantly greater improvement over the controls at 3 months in the area of overall cognitive functioning, psychomotor speed, and verbal learning. No significant difference was observed in work patterns between the 2 groups. Cognitive remediation did not have an effect on symptoms as measured by the PANSS.	Cognitive performance was not measured at the 6- and 12-month follow-ups.
Marder et al. (1996)	Determine the effectiveness of behaviorally social skills training vs. supportive group therapy in supporting the development of social adjustment in participants with schizophrenia	I—Randomized controlled trial *N* = 80 community-dwelling patients with schizophrenia. All had at least 2 acute episodes of schizophrenia or symptoms lasting for at least 2 years. Skills training, *n* = 43 Supportive group therapy, *n* = 37	*Intervention:* Group 1: Behaviorally oriented social skill training group Group 2: Supportive group therapy Both groups participated twice weekly for 6 months and weekly for 18 months. *Outcome Measures:* Social Adjustment Scale II Psychotic exacerbation	Participants in the social skills training group performed significantly better on the total scores of the Social Adjustment Scale II and on the personal well-being subscale. The advantage of social skills group was greatest when combined with active drug supplementation. There was no difference between groups for psychotic exacerbation.	Study participants were all male.

Author/Year	Study Objectives and Design	Intervention and Outcome Measures	Results	Study Limitations
McGrath & Hayes (2000)	Determine whether the use of cognitive rehabilitation techniques is associated with improvement in people with schizophrenia and related conditions I—Systematic review Sample: All relevant randomized controlled studies $N = 3$ studies of individuals with schizophrenia and related conditions	Intervention: Cognitive rehabilitation involved repetitive laboratory-based exercises to train basic-level cognitive processes such as memory, attention, speed of processing, and abstraction levels. Outcome Measures: Studies included in review measured: ■ General level of functioning (e.g., living skills) ■ Mental state (e.g., delusions) ■ Specific cognitive domain (e.g., memory) ■ Quality of life ■ Cost ■ Acceptability of treatment ■ Adverse effects	Evidence inconclusive, with no support for cognitive rehabilitation, placebo, or occupational therapy 3 small studies met the inclusion criteria. 2 compared cognitive rehabilitation with a placebo intervention (total $n = 84$), and 1 with occupational therapy ($n = 33$). Although cognitive rehabilitation was as acceptable as placebo and occupational therapy, with low attrition in both groups, no effects were demonstrated on measures of mental state, social behavior, or cognitive functioning. An effect in favor of cognitive rehabilitation on a measure of self-esteem (Rosenberg Self-Esteem Scale, MD 6.3 CI 1.07–11.53) is worthy of replication in any future trials.	Limited number of studies that were short in duration. Differing measures use in studies.
McGurk, Twamley, Sitzer, McHugo, & Mueser (2007)	Evaluate the effects of cognitive remediation for improving cognitive performance, symptoms, and psychosocial functioning in schizophrenia I—Meta-analysis $N = 26$ randomized controlled trials with 1,151 patients with schizophrenia, schizophreniform disorder or schizoaffective disorder	Intervention: Studies included were of psychosocial interventions designed to improve cognitive performance Outcome Measures: Meta-analysis included studies with at least 1 neuropsychological measure that examined generalization of effects rather than assessment on trained tasks only	The results indicate that there were significant improvements for all outcomes. There were medium effect sizes for cognitive performance and psychosocial functioning and a small effect size for symptoms. The effects of cognitive remediation on psychosocial functioning were stronger for those studies that paired cognitive remediation with psychiatric rehabilitation rather than in those that examined cognitive remediation alone.	Limited number of studies addressing long-term follow-up.

(continued)

Evidence Table 1. Mental Health Recovery Model in the Areas of Community Integration and Normative Life Roles (continued)

Author/Year	Study Objectives	Level/Design/Participants	Intervention and Outcome Measures	Results	Study Limitations
Patterson et al. (2005)	Evaluate the effectiveness of a pilot test of a program for Latino (primarily Mexican) older clients with serious mental illness living mostly with family members	I—Randomized controlled trial N = 29 participants over 40 years old Experimental, n = 21 Control, n = 8	*Intervention:* Programa de Entrenamiento para el Desarollo de Aptitudes para Latinos (PEDAL; Spanish version of the Functional Aptitudes and Skills Training), a 24-wk program of everyday functioning, including social skills, transportation, medication management, communication, and financial management. Control group: Support control condition (supportive environment for discussion of personal problems) *Outcome Measures:* ■ UCSD Performance-Based Skills Assessment (UPSA) ■ Social Skills Performance Assessment (SSPA) Medication Management Abilities Assessment (MMAA) ■ Positive and Negative Syndromes Scale (PANSS) ■ Hamilton Rating Scale for Depression ■ Quality of Well-Being Scale	PEDAL group performed better at 6 months than control on the UPSA ($p < .001$) but was not significantly different at 12 months or 18 months. No significant differences on MMAA or SSPA. Significant difference noted on PANSS at 18 months due to Support Group scoring worse.	At baseline, control group was significantly older than experimental group. Small sample size.
Patterson et al. (2006)	Evaluate a psychosocial intervention designed to improve living skills of older persons with chronic psychotic disorders	I—Randomized controlled trial N = 240 individuals over 40 years old with chronic serious mental illness Functional Adaptation and Skills Training (FAST) group, n = 124 Control group, n = 116	*Intervention:* FAST: Manualized program of everyday functioning, including social skills, medication management, communication, and financial management Control group: Supportive environment for discussion of personal problems *Outcome Measures:* ■ UCSD Performance-based Skills Assessment ■ Social Skills Performance Assessment ■ Medication Management Abilities Assessment ■ Positive and Negative Syndromes Scale ■ Hamilton Rating Scale for Depression ■ Quality of Well-Being Scale	Participants in the FAST program performed better than those in the control group on living skills and social skills but not on medication management.	High dropout rate. Because participants were from board-and-care facilities, the results may not generalize to other populations.

Author (Year)	Study Objective / Design	Intervention / Outcome Measures	Results	Limitations
Tungpunkom & Nicol (2008)	Review the effectiveness of life skills programs with standard care or other comparable programs or therapies for people with chronic mental health problems I—Systematic review *N* = 4 randomized trials Participants: Total of 318 subjects between the ages of 18 and 60 with mental illness. Dementia, substance abuse, alcoholism, organic brain syndrome, and serious suicidal risk were excluded.	*Intervention:* The elements of life skills programs include training in managing money, organizing and running a home, domestic skills, and personal self-care and related interpersonal skills. *Outcome Measures:* Most of the scales used in analysis focused on psychiatric symptoms (mood, depression, positive and negative symptoms) Functional measures Quality of life	This review shows that there is no evidence indicating that such programs are helpful or harmful with respect to functional outcomes and quality of life.	Limited number of randomized controlled studies in this area. Studies included were short-term intervention.
Valencia, Rascon, Juarez, & Murow (2007)	Assess the effectiveness of psychosocial skills training compared with standard treatment in outpatients with chronic schizophrenia in Mexico I—Randomized controlled trial, blinded assessment *N* = 82 (ages 16–50) outpatients with a diagnosis of chronic schizophrenia Treatment as usual (TAU) group, *n* = 39 Intervention group, *n* = 43	*Intervention:* Included TAU plus family therapy and group psychosocial skills sessions of 1 hr and 15 min/wk for 48 wk that focused on 7 treatment areas: symptom management medication management, social relations, occupational therapy, money management, couple relations, and family relations. TAU: 20-min meeting/month with psychiatrist to discuss medication. *Outcome Measures:* ■ Positive and Negative Syndrome Scale ■ Psychosocial Functioning Scale ■ Global Assessment of Functioning Relapse and rehospitalization rates and adherence to medications also were evaluated.	The intervention group demonstrated significant improvement between pre- and postmeasure in the areas of symptomatology, psychosocial functioning, and global functioning as compared with the TAU group. Effect sizes ranged from medium to large for treatment group. In addition, the treatment group had a lower relapse and rehospitalization rate.	Value or benefit of family therapy not discussed or included in statistical models.
Weinhardt, Carey, Carey, & Verdicias (1998)	Examine whether assertiveness training would reduce risk of HIV infection I—Randomized controlled trial *N* = 20 female outpatients with schizophrenia, bipolar disorder, or major depressive disorder Intervention group, *n* = 9 Wait list control group, *n* = 11	*Intervention:* 3 sessions on HIV-related information; remainder of sessions focused on sexual assertiveness training on initiating discussion, negotiation, and refusing to engage in unsafe sex; used modeling, simulation, practice and feedback. *Outcome Measures:* ■ Sexual Assertiveness Simulation ■ HIV-Knowledge Questionnaire ■ Perceived Risk Questionnaire ■ Behavioral Intentions Questionnaire ■ Timeline Followback Sexual Behavior Interview ■ Treatment Acceptability Questionnaire	Significant differences in assertiveness skill ($p < .001$) and HIV knowledge ($p < .001$) at postintervention and most 4-month follow-ups for intervention group. There was no difference between groups on motivation indexes of perceived risk and behavioral intentions. Condom use did not differ at 4-month follow-up.	Small sample size; absence of attention control group.

(continued)

Evidence Table 1. Mental Health Recovery Model in the Areas of Community Integration and Normative Life Roles (continued)

Author/Year	Study Objectives	Level/Design/Participants	Intervention and Outcome Measures	Results	Study Limitations
Wykes, Reeder, Corner, Williams, & Everitt (1999)	Evaluate the effectiveness of a neurocognitive training program	I—Randomized controlled trial $N = 33$ persons with schizophrenia Neurocognitive remediation (NCR) group, $n = 17$ Intensive occupational therapy control group, $n = 16$	*Intervention:* NCR is a manualized daily program for complex planning and problem solving and included fine motor, perceptual–motor, and conceptual tasks. Control group: Intensive occupational therapy *Outcome Measures:* ■ Cognitive flexibility ■ Planning ■ Memory and working memory ■ Functional measures ■ Symptoms and social functioning	Participants in the NCR group had significantly more improvement on cognitive flexibility, memory, and self-esteem, but there were no differences between groups on other scores.	Small sample size; question of group equivalence.
Wykes et al. (2003)	Evaluate the effectiveness of a cognitive remediation training program at 6-month follow-up	I—Randomized controlled trial $N = 33$ persons with schizophrenia Neurocognitive remediation (NCR) group, $n = 17$ Intensive occupational therapy control group, $n = 16$	*Intervention:* NCR is a manualized daily program for complex planning and problem solving and included fine motor, perceptual–motor, and conceptual tasks. Control group: Intensive occupational therapy *Outcome Measures:* ■ Cognitive flexibility ■ Planning ■ Memory and working memory ■ Functional measures ■ Symptoms and social functioning	Changes in memory still evident at 6-month follow-up, although not for self-esteem.	Small sample size; question of group equivalence.
Xia & Li (2007)	Review the effectiveness of problem-solving therapy compared with other comparable therapies or routine care for persons with schizophrenia	I—Systematic review $N = 3$ randomized controlled trials with a total of 52 participants	*Intervention:* Compared problem-solving therapy with routine care, coping skills training, or nonspecific intervention. Therapy interventions done by psychiatrists, psychologists, registered nurses, and general practitioners; supportive therapies. *Outcome Measures:* ■ Behavior and social skills ■ Mental state	No differences found between groups; authors reported that results are insufficient due to limitations of studies included in review.	Small study sizes; poor data reporting; measures unsuitable for data analysis; studies reported being randomized, but randomization was not discussed in studies.

Level II

Bartels et al. (2004)	Assess the effectiveness of a combined skills training (ST) and health management intervention (HM) for older adults with severe mental illness	II—Nonrandomized controlled trial

N = 24 persons ages 60 or older with a diagnosis of schizophrenia, schizoaffective disorder, bipolar disorder, other psychotic disorder or treatment refractory depression and persistent functional impairment requiring ongoing support
HM+ST (intervention), n = 12
HM only (control), n = 12 | *Intervention:*
ST: Hourlong group skills training 2×/wk adapted from manualized skills training programs delivered by a nurse case manager. HM: Assessment and monitoring of routine and chronic health care needs and promotion of preventive health care. Delivered by same nurse case manager.
Intervention Group: HM+ST
Control Group: HM

Outcome Measures:
- Independent Living Skills Survey
- Social Behavior Schedule
- Brief Psychiatric Rating Scale
- Scale for the Assessment of Negative Symptoms
- Geriatric Depression Scale
- Mini Mental State Exam Preventive health care | After 1 year, the HM+ST group had better functional outcomes, with medium to large effect sizes with respect to independent living skills, social skills, and health management, compared to those receiving HM alone. After 2 years, both groups had improved preventive health care. | Lack of randomization; pilot study had a small sample size. |
| Bickes, DeLoache, Dicer, & Miller (2001) | Examine the effectiveness of occupation-based verbal therapy vs. occupation-based experiential therapy on the money management skills of consumers of community mental health services | II—Nonrandomized controlled trial

N = 14 consumers from a community mental health day support program.

Diagnoses included schizophrenia, personality disorders, and mood disorders. | *Intervention:*
COPM was administered to determine which occupation clients were most interested in. Clients identified money management.
Group 1: Occupation-based experiential group
Group 2: Verbal group
Occupational therapy groups conducted 3×/wk for 2 wk by 2 certified occupational therapy assistant students.

Outcome Measures:
- Comprehensive Occupational Therapy Evaluation (COTE)
- Milwaukee Evaluation of Daily Living Skills (MEDLS) | There was no significant difference between the verbal group and the experiential group on the COTE or on the MEDLS. Overall performance of both groups improved significantly on the COTE, but did not improve significantly on the MEDLS. | Short time frame of intervention may have been inadequate to allow for experiential learning to occur.

Small sample size; lack of control group.

Experiential groups occurred in simulated environment instead of community. |

(continued)

Evidence Table 1. Mental Health Recovery Model in the Areas of Community Integration and Normative Life Roles (continued)

Author/Year	Study Objectives	Level/Design/Participants	Intervention and Outcome Measures	Results	Study Limitations
Brown, Goetz, Van Sciver, Sullivan, & Hamera (2006)	Examine the efficacy of a psychiatric rehabilitation weight loss program	II—Nonrandomized controlled trial N = 36 participants from a support program for people with psychiatric disabilities with a BMI ≥ 25 Experimental group, n = 21 Control group, n = 15	*Intervention:* Experimental: 12-wk manualized intervention combining evidence-based weight loss and psychiatric rehabilitation strategies Control group: Participants recruited after start on experimental group; no intervention provided *Outcome Measures:* • Body weight • BMI • Waist circumference • Blood pressure • Health Promoting Lifestyle Profile II	At follow-up, the intervention group improved significantly on body weight, BMI, waist circumference, and the physical activity subscale of the Health Promoting Lifestyle Profile II. The intervention group lost 6 lbs, and the control group gained 1 lb. There were no differences between groups at follow-up for blood pressure, total, and nutrition subscale of the Health Promoting Lifestyle II.	Small sample size; lack of randomization.
Hutchinson, Skrinar, & Cross (1999)	Evaluate the effect of aerobic exercise on recovery of adults with severe mental illness (bipolar disorders, schizophrenia, personality disorders)	II—2-part quasi-experimental design Part 1 was modified time series (reporting on 2 sets of multiple groupings); Part 2 was pretest–posttest with randomization Exercise group, n = 37 Comparison group, n = 6	*Intervention:* Exercise class met 3×/wk for 1 hr in early afternoon, for either 20 or 15 wk. After class completion, participants were assigned to either support (encouraging follow-up exercises) or nonsupport groups. Comparison group: No intervention. *Outcome Measures:* ■ Physiological measures Exercise Tolerance Test (ETT) ■ Tennessee Self-Concept Scale ■ Beck Depression Inventory	No precise statistics reported. Reported as significant: Participants who exercised over time experienced an overall rise in self-esteem; exercise had antidepressant effect; performance times on ETT improved. Although participants reported increases in ADLs performance and satisfaction, those changes were not significant. No differences noted in follow-up part of experiment.	Participant numbers not consistent for evaluation of attrition, although reported approximately 20% for each group. Lack of clear statistical reporting; small comparison group.
Kelley, Coursey, & Selby (1997)	Examine the effectiveness of outdoor adventure programs to improve function in persons with serious mental illness	Level III—Multiple group pretest/posttest design N = 57 with schizophrenia, affective disorders Intervention group, n = 38 Control, n = 19	*Intervention:* Outdoor activities plus self-instruction training Control group: Did not consent to participate in program *Outcome Measures:* Generalized Self-Efficacy Scale ■ Self-Efficacy Scale ■ Perceived Physical Ability and Physical Self-Presentation Confidence subscales of the Physical Self-Efficacy Scale ■ Rosenberg Self-Esteem Inventory ■ State–Trait Anxiety Inventory ■ Beck Depression Inventory ■ Anxiety and Depression subscales of the Brief Symptom Inventory ■ Trust & Cooperation Scale ■ Internal Locus of Control ■ Global Severity Index	Participants in the outdoor adventure group showed significant improvement in self-efficacy and self-esteem compared with the controls. Decreases in anxiety and depression were observed on some measures (Brief Symptom Inventory) but not on others. There were no effects on locus of control.	The quasi-experimental design presented several threats to internal validity, such as selection × maturation effects. However, experimental vs. control differences were not found at pretest, and adventure group participants showed no significant changes between the first and second (the wait list period) pretests. The use of dropouts as controls (done to increase N and thus power) may be questionable.

Citation	Study Objective/Design/Participants	Intervention and Outcome Measures	Results	Study Limitations
Leclerc, Lesage, Ricard, Lecomte, & Cyr (2000)	Determine the effectiveness of a the Coping Skills Module for persons with schizophrenia II—Nonrandomized controlled trial $N = 99$ persons with schizophrenia randomly drawn from 3 different pools. Intervention group, $n = 36$ Treatment as usual (TAU), $n = 44$ Those who dropped out of intervention (15 men, 4 women) were allocated to an intent-to-treat group.	*Intervention:* The treatment group received regular rehabilitation treatment (TAU) plus a coping skills module that included problem solving and cognitive behavior therapy. *Outcome Measures:* • Interview • French version of the Positive and Negative Syndrome Scale • Independent Living Skills Scale • French version of the Rosenberg Self-Esteem Scale • French version of the Stress Appraisal Measure • Cybernetic Coping Scale	Participants in the coping skills group were significantly more likely than controls to experience a decrease in delusions and an increase in self-esteem at the 6-month follow-up. The experimental group maintained levels of hygiene, while the control group experienced a significant decline in hygiene at follow-up. Stress appraisal, coping, and reappraisal, the process variable directly targeted by the intervention, did not show significant differences across groups over time; neither did they act as covariates.	More women than men participated in the experimental group than the control group. Three-quarters of participants were living in a psychiatric hospital during treatment.
Moriana, Alarcon, & Herruzo (2006)	Determine the outcomes/effectiveness of a social and independent living skills intervention developed by Liberman, Wallace, Blackwell, Kopelowicz, Vaccaro, and Mintz (1998) provided in an in-home setting in Spain. II—Nonrandomized controlled trial $N = 64$ participants with schizophrenia recruited from a mental health facility in Spain. All patients were receiving outpatient psychiatric treatment and neuroleptics $n = 32$ in each group	*Intervention:* In-home social and independent living skills program including the following components: medication and symptom management, recreation for leisure, basic conversational skills, and community reentry. Control: Participants attended day treatment program. *Outcome Measures:* Positive and Negative Symptom Scale (PANSS)	There was a significant phase-by-treatment interaction effect for the intervention on PANSS scores.	Limited outcome measures; lack of randomization. Very expensive to carry out because of the intensity of the contacts.
Patterson et al. (2003)	Evaluate the efficacy of a skills training program to improve functioning in middle-age and older adults with chronic psychotic disorders I—Randomized controlled trial $N = 40$ patients at board-and-care facility Intervention group, $n = 16$ Control group, $n = 16$ (8 dropouts)	*Intervention:* 24 sessions of Functional Adaptation Skills Training (FAST), a manualized social–cognitive theory–based behavioral intervention focused on improving medication management, social skills, communication skill, organization and planning, transportation, and financial management Control: Treatment as usual *Outcome Measures:* • UCSD Performance-Based Skills Assessment: Functional skills • Positive and Negative Syndromes Scales • Hamilton Rating Scale for Depression • Quality of Well-Being Scale	Functional performance following participation in the FAST program improved significantly postintervention and was maintained at 3-month follow-up in comparison to control group. There was no change in psychopathology during the treatment and follow-up periods.	Performance-based functional measure may not accurately portray real-life performance. Client contact was greater for FAST than for the control condition, which may explain the differences in results.

(continued)

Evidence Table 1. Mental Health Recovery Model in the Areas of Community Integration and Normative Life Roles (*continued*)

Author/Year	Study Objectives	Level/Design/Participants	Intervention and Outcome Measures	Results	Study Limitations
Roder et al. (2002)	Evaluate the effect of cognitive social skills training programs on cognitive and social abilities, psychopathology, and generalization effects	II—Nonrandomized intervention comparison of 3 specific programs vs. control of general social skills training and problem-solving training N = 105 n = 73 in 3 experimental groups n = 32 control participants with schizophrenia or schizoaffective disorder	*Intervention:* Three specific cognitive social skills programs (residential, vocational, or recreational) Control condition: General social skills training *Outcome Measures:* ■ Number Connecting Test ■ Continuous Concentration Test ■ Attention–Stress Test ■ Global Assessment of Functioning ■ Social Interview Schedule ■ Disability Assessment Schedule ■ Intentionality Rating Scale Brief Psychiatric Rating Scale ■ Scale for the Assessment of Negative Symptoms Scale for the Assessment of Well-Being	Higher global therapy effects were found for nearly all dependent variables in the 3 cognitive social skills groups. All effects indicated improvement in aftercare and follow-up phase. There was more relapse in control participants than experimental participants 48 wk after beginning therapy. There were significantly greater improvements in the control group on cognitive factors.	Groups not equivalent at baseline and not randomized.
Schindler (1999)	Examine the effectiveness of an activity group, structured discussion, and control group for social interaction skills of persons with psychiatric disabilities	II—Nonrandomized controlled trial N = 25 participants with severe psychiatric disability Structured discussion group, n = 9 Activity group, n = 6 Control group, n = 10	*Intervention:* Activity group: Guided purposeful tasks to provide a focus for skill development Structured verbal discussion: Set topic or agenda (e.g., use of leisure time) Control group: Provided with table games All took place 5×/wk for 2 wk *Outcome Measures:* ■ Global Assessment Scale ■ Social Functioning Index	The activity group showed a significant improvement in social interaction skills as compared to the structured verbal discussion and control groups.	Small sample size; other activities may have been taking place during study period.
Schindler (2005)	Examine whether adults diagnosed with schizophrenia demonstrated improved task and interpersonal skills and social roles when involved in a individualized intervention based on the Role Development Program (RDP), in comparison to an intervention based on a multidepartmental activity program (MAP)	II—Nonrandomized controlled trial N = 84 participants, 42 per group, all male with diagnosis of schizophrenia disorder	*Intervention:* Group 1 (comparison): MAP—a non-individualized, therapeutic intervention designed to encourage the productive use of time and socialization in a group setting. Does not address social roles or skills imbedded in social roles. Group 2 (experimental): RDP—an enhancement of the MAP. Utilizes individualized theory-based interventions to help each participant develop task and interpersonal skills within meaningful social roles. Frequency: Both groups received 15 min/wk of individual attention. Other meeting times were not reported. Duration varied from 4, 8, and 12 wk. *Outcome Measures:* ■ Role Functioning Scale ■ Task Skills Scale ■ Interpersonal Skills Scale	Participants in the RDP demonstrated greater improvement in social roles, task skills, and interpersonal skills than participants in the MAP.	Results may not generalize to individuals in other treatment settings. Staff involved in the RDP may not be typical of staff in other treatment settings. Full validity studies had not been conducted on 2 of the assessment instruments.

Study	Study Objectives	Level/Design	Intervention and Outcome Measures	Results	Study Limitations
Wong-McDonald (2007)	Examine whether the inclusion of a spiritual-ity group enhances the recovery of persons participating in psychiatric rehabilitation program	II—Nonrandomized controlled trial $N = 48$ individuals who were attending a psychiatric rehabilitation program with at least 50% attendance for at least 3 months Spirituality group (SG) in addition to the required skills training program, $n = 20$ Control group, $n = 28$	*Intervention:* SG was a weekly 60-min optional session in a psychiatric rehabilitation program focusing on skills training. SG group was conducted with a focus on group members' definitions of spirituality to empower participants toward recovery through spiritual pathways. The group used spiritual music and writings, with topics of discussion such as forgiveness, love, and self-worth. *Outcome Measures:* Number of treatment goals achieved	All 20 participants (100%) in the SG achieved their treatment goals, compared with 16 of 28 (57%) control participants. The difference in goal attainment between the 2 groups was significant with the Fisher exact one-tailed test ($p = .0001$). Chi-square results were not significant.	Small group size; lack of randomization.
Wu (2001)	Examine effectiveness of an occupational therapy intervention to facilitate intrinsic motivation in persons with psychiatric illness and difficulties with motivation	II—Mixed-effects nested design (2-group control) Participants were clients from 3 general hospital psychiatric units, and 3 psychiatric hospitals in Taiwan $N = 99$ participants from initial 166 volunteers	*Intervention:* Intervention was an occupational therapist providing structured experiences for success and providing an intervention environment that promoted choice/autonomy for 12 wk. Control: Occupational therapy treatment as usual for 12 wk. *Outcome Measures:* ■ Chinese Comprehensive Occupational Therapy Evaluation (COTE) ■ Chinese General Causality Orientations Scale ■ Pearson product moment for comparing intrinsic motivation and behavioral change	There was a significant improvement in motivation in the experimental group who had motivation deficits as compared to the control group. The improvement in intrinsic motivation was correlated with change in observed social behavior. The mixed-type participants did not gain significant benefit from the motivational intervention.	Author reports that outcome measures have some psychometric limitations.

Level III

Briand et al. (2006)	Assess the clinical outcomes of adding Integrated Psychological Treatment (IPT) to standard care in adults with schizophrenia in Canada	III—One-group, multisite pretest/posttest design $N = 90$; 55 participants completed the program. 23 of the 26 mental health professionals implementing this program were occupational therapists.	*Intervention:* IPT is a cognitive behavioral group program consisting of 6 subprograms of exercises that increase in complexity over the 6 months of implementation. *Outcome Measures:* ■ Frankfurt Complaint Questionnaire–short version ■ Client's Assessment of Strengths, Interests, and Goals–Self-Report ■ Client's Assessment of Strengths, Interests, and Goals–Informant Version, Symptoms Section ■ Multnomah Community Ability Scales ■ Structured Clinical Interview for *DSM–IV* ■ Cambridge Neuropsychological Test Automated Battery	Including IPT with standard medical therapy was associated with statistically significant positive clinical outcomes across time in overall symptoms, subjective experiences, cognitive and social functioning, and quality of life. Positive effects on symptomatology were noticed early (after first 3 modules). Long-term effects varied from site to site. Effects for social functioning and quality of life took longer to integrate.	Lack of control group.

(continued)

Evidence Table 1. Mental Health Recovery Model in the Areas of Community Integration and Normative Life Roles (continued)

Author/Year	Study Objectives	Level/Design/Participants	Intervention and Outcome Measures	Results	Study Limitations
Cook et al. (2010)	Evaluate the outcomes of statewide initiatives to teach self-management of mental illness to people in a peer-led self-management program in mental health recovery	III—Pretest/posttest design N = 381 participants in a peer-led self-management program in Vermont and Minnesota	*Intervention:* Wellness Recovery Action Planning (WRAP), in which participants identify internal and external resources for facilitating recovery and use these tools to create an individualized plan *Outcome Measures:* Surveys developed in 2 WRAP programs to evaluate attitudes such as hope for recovery and responsibility for wellness, knowledge of early warning signs for decompensation, symptom triggers, use of skills, and wellness tools	Significant changes were observed in both WRAP programs on posttest in hopefulness for recovery, warning signs of decompensation, use of wellness tools, awareness of symptom triggers, having a crisis plan and a plan for dealing with symptoms, having a social support system, and the ability to take responsibility for wellness.	2 programs used slightly different outcome measures. No follow-up after the completion of the program. Survey measure has not been tested. Lack of control group.
Eklund (2001)	Evaluate occupational roles following a period of occupational therapy followed by a 1-year follow-up	III—Pretest/posttest design N = 20-day hospital patients	*Intervention:* Individual and group occupational therapy provided 20 hr/wk over a period of 4 days in a day-care unit. *Outcome Measures:* ■ Role Checklist (Swedish version) ■ Self-rating subjective quality of life ■ Health-Sickness Rating Scale	The number of valued roles increased significantly from admission to discharge and follow-up. 5 of 8 valued roles, friend, hobbyist, worker, family member, and caregiver showed associations with quality of life, and the relationship of friend to quality of life was most consistent over the 3 measurement points. No association was found between occupational roles and a general measure of mental health.	Lack of control group.
Halford, Harrison, Kalysnsundaram, Moutrey, & Simpson (1995)	Conduct a preliminary study of the effectiveness of a psychoeducational program to rehabilitate chronic patients to improve community functioning	III—Pretest/posttest design N = 22 clients with schizophrenia or affective disorder with psychotic features Age range: 26–50 years	*Intervention:* Provided structured skills training consisting of 5 14-wk modules focused on medication and symptom self-management, coping with anxiety and depression, social skills, living skills, and leisure skills. *Outcome Measures:* ■ Brief Psychiatric Rating Scale ■ Quality of Life Scale ■ Scale for the Assessment of Negative Symptoms ■ Life Skills Profile	Participants improved significantly on all measures except for the Life Skills Profile.	Small sample size; high dropout rate from program. A large number of participants did not complete the Life Skills Profile.

Author (Year)	Study Objective	Level of Evidence/Design/Sample	Intervention and Outcome Measures	Results	Study Limitations
Helfrich, Aviles, Badiani, Walens, & Sabol (2006)	Evaluate the effectiveness of interventions focusing on skills specific to each of 3 groups of homeless individuals: youth without families (employment skills), women fleeing abusive homes (managing finances), and persons with mental illnesses (securing and managing food)	III—Three-group pretest/posttest design $N = 73$ Age range: 17–55 years; 63 female, 10 male; 72% were youth Adults with mental illness, $n = 13$ Domestic violence victims, $n = 13$ Youth, $n = 6$	*Intervention:* Group life skills sessions and individual sessions, each 1×/wk for 4 consecutive weeks based on MOHO. The focus of the intervention for adults with mental illness was on food and nutrition with group session goals and individual goals for each member. *Outcome Measures:* Ansell–Casey Life Skill Assessment and Quiz	20 participants increased their mastery scores, 5 demonstrated no change in scores, and 7 demonstrated a decrease in scores. Although women experiencing domestic violence had a significant improvement on life skill scores, there were no statically significant changes in the youth group or group with mental illness.	Groups were small and diverse in abilities, backgrounds, education and skills. Only 1 test used for outcome measures. Quantitative outcomes were limited in generalizability. Difficulty retaining participants due to transience of populations.
Helfrich, Chan, & Sabol (2011)	Evaluate the effectiveness of a life skills intervention for adults with mental illness who have been homeless	III—Pretest/posttest design $N = 38$ adults with documented mental illness recruited either from an emergency housing program or single-room occupancy program	*Intervention:* Life skills intervention consisted of 4 modules: (1) room and self-care management, (2) food management, (3) money management, and (4) safe community participation. *Outcome Measures:* ■ Allen Cognitive Level Screen 2000 (ACLS–2000) ■ Practical Skills Test (PST)	The PST scores of participants with higher ACLS–2000 scores significantly increased over time for food management, money management, and safe community participation. Those with lower ACLS–2000 scores had an even greater change over time.	Small sample size; narrow range of diagnostic categories and cognitive levels. Although a small control group ($n = 8$) was initially included, it was eliminated from the analysis.
Phelan, Lee, Howe, & Walter (2006)	Describe a pilot group program in Australia for parents with a mental illness	III—Pretest/posttest design $N = 29$ parents; 19 completed the program	*Intervention:* The Parenting and Mental Illness Group Program consisted of a 6-wk group program followed by 4 individual follow-up sessions. Interviews were conducted at intake. *Outcome Measures:* ■ Eyberg Child Behaviour Inventory ■ Parenting Scale	At posttest, 40% fewer parents were in the "intensity" clinical range, and 57% fewer were in the "problem" range on the Eyberg. On the Parenting Scale, 26% fewer were in the clinical range for laxness, 45% for overreactivity, and 33% for verbosity.	Small sample size; attrition from program at completion and completion of posttest; no comparison statistics were included.
Stein, Cislo, & Ward (1994)	Evaluate a 1-semester practicum course on social relationships to demonstrate benefit of clinic/community sharing of resources	III—2-group pretest/posttest design $N = 14$ people with psychiatric disability and 14 college undergraduates, plus nonequivalent control groups for each experimental group	*Intervention:* Participation in 2×/wk class for 15 wk (1 didactic, 1 structured exercises [problem solving, discussion] per week). Pairing of community residents and undergraduate students who also met outside class to do homework. *Outcome Measures:* ■ Personal Network Interview ■ Interpersonal Self-Efficacy Index ■ Social Response Questionnaire ■ Perception of Relationship Change ■ Behavior Assertiveness Test–Revised	Community-dwelling students (persons with a psychiatric disability) reported a significant increase in feelings of interpersonal self-efficacy ($p < .001$). There were few significant main effects, but there were reported and observed positive changes in social functioning (nonverbal behavior, interpersonal assertiveness and skills behaviors) compared with control participants.	Exact number of experimental cohort participants was questionable (some attrition noted). Small sample sizes reduce possibility of statistical the significance. Ceiling effect in many measures for undergraduate students.

(continued)

Evidence Table 1. Mental Health Recovery Model in the Areas of Community Integration and Normative Life Roles (*continued*)

Author/Year	Study Objectives	Level/Design/Participants	Intervention and Outcome Measures	Results	Study Limitations
Starino et al. (2010)	Examine the effect of participating in an illness self-management recovery program on the ability of participants with severe mental illness to achieve key recovery-related outcomes	III—Pretest/posttest design *N* = 30 adults with severe mental illness at 3 mental health centers in the Midwest	*Intervention:* Participation in a WRAP group, peer-led sessions that focus on wellness tools, creating a list of daily maintenance activities, identifying illness triggers and early warning signs, and developing a crisis plan. *Outcome Measures:* ▪ State Hope Scale ▪ Modified Colorado Symptom Index ▪ Recovery Markers Questionnaire	A significant positive time effect was found for hope and recovery orientation. The change in symptoms did not reach statistical significance.	Small sample size, lack of control group, limited follow-up period.

Note. ADLs = activities of daily living; ANOVA = analysis of variance; BMI = body mass index; COPM = Canadian Occupational Performance Measure; *DSM–IV* = *Diagnostic and Statistical Manual of Mental Disorders, 4th Edition;* MOHO = Model of Human Occupation; UCLA = University of California, Los Angeles; UCSD = University of California, San Diego.

Evidence Table 2. Mental Health—Paid and Unpaid Employment and Education

Author/Year	Study Objectives	Level/Design/Participants	Intervention and Outcome Measures	Results	Study Limitations
Level I					
Anzai, Yoneda, Nakamura, Ikebuchi, & Liberman (2002)	Examine the effectiveness of the Community Re-Entry Module skills training program when adapted for Japanese psychiatric patients in teaching knowledge and skills required to live and participate in the community	I—Randomized controlled trial $N = 29$ participants diagnosed with schizophrenia Group 1: $n = 14$ Group 2: $n = 15$ Mean duration of illness: 20.5 years Mean duration of hospitalization: 4 years Mean age: 46.8 years	*Intervention* Group 1, Community Re-entry Module: Highly structured curriculum that consists of sessions on medication, relapse, finding housing and psychiatric care in the community, reducing stress and coping Group 2, control—Conventional occupational rehabilitation program, consisting of arts and crafts, reality orientation groups, and work assignments in the hospital Who delivered: Groups 1 and 2: Ward nurse Frequency/duration: Groups 1 and 2: 18 1-hr sessions 2×/wk *Outcome Measures:* ■ Hospital discharge rates ■ Rehabilitation Evaluation Hall and Baker (REHAB) scale, a 23-item tool that measures self-care, social, and independent living skills ■ A 21-item instrument that is part of the Community Re-entry Module and measures skills addressed in the module	Group 1 demonstrated significantly higher scores on the Community Re-entry Module 21-item instrument at a 1-year follow-up, whereas Group 2 did not. Group 1 demonstrated significantly better improvement in skills measured by the REHAB scale, whereas Group 2 did not.	The Community Re-entry Module was modified for clients in Japanese psychiatric care. The results may not generalize to U.S. health care systems; however, the module was adapted from the Community Re-entry Module that was designed and validated by associates at the UCLA psychiatric rehabilitation program. No comparison between groups was reported.

(continued)

Evidence Table 2. Mental Health—Paid and Unpaid Employment and Education (continued)

Author/Year	Study Objectives	Level/Design/Participants	Intervention and Outcome Measures	Results	Study Limitations
Bell, Bryson, Greig, Corcoran, & Wexler (2001)	Evaluate the effects of neurocognitive enhancement therapy (NET) in combination with work therapy (WT) on performance on neuropsychological tests.	I—Randomized controlled trial N = 65 participants with schizophrenia or schizoaffective disorder Random assignment to NET + WT (n = 31) or WT only (n = 34)	*Intervention:* WT consisted of payment for work, job placement, individual counseling, support group, Work Behavior Inventory feedback, job coach, participation certificate and vocational services referral. NET: feedback from Cognitive Functional Assessment, cognitive exercises for up to 5 hours/wk for 26 wk, and a weekly social processing group. Cognitive exercises involved repeated practice on computer-based exercises for attention, memory, and executive function *Outcome Measures:* ■ Neuropsychological testing: portions of Wechsler Adult Intelligence Scale–II (WAIS–II) and Wechsler Memory Scale–Revised (WMS–R); Hopkins Verbal Learning Test (HVLT), Continuous Performance Test, Wisconsin Card Sorting Test (WCST); Bell Lysaker Emotion Recognition Task (BLERT); Gorham's Proverbs Test; Hinting task; Trail-Making Test–B. ■ Work performance: Work Behavior Inventory; Work Personality Profile ■ Cognitive Functional Assessment scale ■ Positive and Negative Syndrome Scale	Overall, the results indicate significant improvements in neuropsychological functioning for the NET + WT group. Affect recognition and working memory improved more for the NET + WT clients. For this group the percent of normal scores on the BLERT increased from 35%–60% compared to a decline for WT-only clients. Similarly, normal scores on the Digit Span Backward increased from 45%–77% for the NET + WT group compared to a decline for the WT-only group. NET + WT led to greater improvement in executive functioning. Normal conceptual level responses increased from 39%–48% for the NET + WT compared to 29%–42% for WT. Clients with nonperseverative error within the normal range improved 45%–52% for NET + WT clients and decreased slightly for WT clients. Tasks sensitive to conceptual and language disorganization and verbal/nonverbal secondary memory tasks did not show differential improvement for NET + WT.	This study did not control for the amount of productive activity clients could engage in; did not include a no treatment control group; imaging studies were not performed that would have helped determine how NET + WT may have affected brain function or structure.
Bell, Fiszdon, Greig, & Bryson (2005)	Compare whether older people with schizophrenia or schizoaffective disorder can benefit from work therapy as well as their younger counterparts	I—Randomized controlled trial Participants were in treatment at the VA Medical Center, West Haven, CT, or at the Connecticut Mental Health Center. N = 145. 41 were >50 years of age (M = 53.3, range: 50–58). Participants were stratified on the basis of work experience and randomly assigned to neurocognitive enhancement treatment plus work therapy or work therapy only.	*Intervention:* Same as Bell et al. (2001). Biweekly assessments of work performance for 6 months for a total of 13 observations *Outcome Measures:* ■ Neuropsychological testing: Portions of Wechsler Adult Intelligence Scale–II (WAIS–II) and Wechsler Memory Scale–Revised (WMS–R); Hopkins Verbal Learning Test (HVLT), Continuous Performance Test, Wisconsin Card Sorting Task (WCST), Bell Lysaker Emotion Recognition Task (BLERT), Gorham's Proverbs Test, Hinting task; Trail-Making Test–B ■ Work performance: Work Behavior Inventory, Work Personality Profile, Cognitive Functional Assessment Scale, Positive and Negative Syndrome Scale	Overall results indicated that older people benefit clinically and vocationally from work rehabilitation as much as their younger counterparts. The older group performed worse than the younger group on executive functioning (cognitive inflexibility, disinhibition, and poor affect recognition) tasks; however, the outcome measures were not age-corrected and may not indicate that the older participants declined more quickly than younger ones. Scores on the PANSS and Quality of Life Scale (QLS) showed a significant time effect with both age groups, but no group effect or Group 3 Time interaction. Both groups improved in work performance over time. Younger workers plateaued in performance in the second 13 wk, whereas older workers continued to improve.	Lack of a no-work control group; limited age range for older sample.

		Intervention:	The WBI group showed significant improvement on personal presentation, social skills, cooperativeness, and total WBI score as compared with participants in the usual support condition. The WBI participants worked significantly more hours than those in the usual supports group.	Study done with men only in late 40s; the usual support group was still within the transitional work program, so supports were more than if control group consisted of participants in competitive work; limited follow-up period.
Bell, Lysaker, & Bryson (2003)	Determine whether work performance feedback from the Work Behavior Inventory (WBI), along with goal setting, improves performance compared with usual supports	I—Randomized controlled trial

$N = 122$ veterans with a diagnosis of schizophrenia or schizoaffective disorders in a stable phase of the disorder and no housing changes

Exclusion criteria: traumatic brain injury, developmental disabilities, or neurological disease. Participants were randomized to the WBI group or usual supports and were stratified according to work experience and negative symptoms. They were then randomly assigned to paid or unpaid work. After excluding those who declined unpaid work or worked longer than 3 wk, 63 participants remained.

WBI group: $n = 30$, mean age: 44.4 years
Usual supports group: $n = 33$; mean age: 43.6 years | Participants were offered a 26-wk job in medical records, escorting, mailroom, dietetics, engineering, and maintenance.
WBI group: The WBI evaluations were completed weekly, starting with Week 1 through observation and supervisor interviews. A group of 6 received WBI feedback for 60 min 1×/wk on items that raised or lowered their score. A goal was set each week that was written on their time sheets. A new goal was written after completion of previous goal.
Control group: Usual support.

Outcome Measures:
- WBI, 5 scales (Work Habits, Work Quality, Personal Presentation, Cooperativeness, Social Skills)
- Positive and Negative Syndrome Scale
- Quality of Life Scale | |
| | | | | The study did not blind the raters; the raters were aware of conditions, and this may have affected ratings. |
| Bond, Drake, & Becker (2008) | Evaluate the effectiveness of the Individual Placement and Support Model (IPS) of supported employment, limiting the review to those studies that have high fidelity to the program | I—Systematic review

Randomized controlled studies from published systematic reviews, review of studies included in the Employment Intervention Demonstration Project, contact with primary investigators or study, and continuous review of the literature | This updated systematic review examined longitudinal competitive employment, one of which used a high-fidelity IPS supported employment model. Control group or groups must have received either services as usual or some other form of vocational rehabilitation besides IPS.

Outcome Measures:
Employment rates, days to first job, annualized weeks worked, and job tenure in longest job held during the follow-up period | The results of this review of 11 studies are consistent with earlier reviews but somewhat stronger due to the high fidelity of the IPS model.

The competitive employment rate was 61% for IPS compared to 23% for controls. Two-thirds of those in competitive employment worked 20 hr or more per week, and their first job was obtained almost 10 wk earlier than did controls. For those in competitive employment, duration of job was approximately one-half year. | Lack of standardization in follow-up periods; relatively short follow-up period. |

(continued)

Evidence Table 2. Mental Health—Paid and Unpaid Employment and Education *(continued)*

Author/Year	Study Objectives	Level/Design/Participants	Intervention and Outcome Measures	Results	Study Limitations
Collins, Bybee, & Mowbray (1998)	Evaluate the effectiveness of 3 supported education program models	I—Randomized controlled trial N = 397; 135 in classroom condition, 134 in group, 128 in individual Participants were recruited through Detroit mental health services with (1) a psychiatric disorder for at least 1 year; (2) high school diploma or GED nearly completed; (3) interest in secondary education; and (4) willing to use mental health services if needed.	*Intervention:* Participants received 2-hour orientation and randomly assigned to 1 of 3 conditions: classroom, group, or individual. Classroom: In 14-wk semesters, 2.5-hr sessions 2×/wk with academic supported curriculum with 3 objectives: managing campus, career exploration, stress management. Group: Aim to support learning environment to explore career or education choices. 2 facilitators helped with use of educational resources. Individual: Control group. No structure or scheduled intervention. Participants assigned to staff to assist for own needs. *Outcome Measures:* ▪ Participation level in program ▪ Involvement in employment, school/vocational program ▪ Motivation, satisfaction, enjoyment level, learning, empowerment, and self-efficacy	At graduation from the program, group members had the highest level of participation, followed by classroom and individual. For the immediate outcomes of motivation, satisfaction, enjoyment, and learning, those who had highest levels of participation had the best outcomes on these measures. For the intermediate outcomes of empowerment and self-efficacy, those in the classroom condition scored significantly higher than those in the group, then individual. While there were no differences in later involvement in jobs or school by condition, the number enrolled in educational or vocational programs was twice that at baseline.	High dropout rate. Results were taken only from those whose completed graduation; therefore, results on outcomes may differ if those who dropped out were interviewed. Information regarding reasons for dropping out may also be investigated.
Cook et al. (2005)	Evaluate the effect of supported employment (SE) on achieving competitive employment for persons with severe mental illness	I—Randomized controlled trial, multisite N = 1,273 8 study sites in Maryland, Connecticut, South Carolina, Pennsylvania, Arizona, Massachusetts, Maine, and Texas were chosen through the Employment Intervention Demonstration Program. Participants at each site were randomly assigned to the SE intervention or the control condition.	*Intervention* All SE sites included integrated multidisciplinary services 3×/wk to plan employment interventions, placement into competitive employment, development of jobs that matched clients' preferences, immediate job search at clients' pace, and ongoing vocational support. Clinical services included psychiatric evaluation; medication management; individual, family, or couples' counseling; case management; and psychosocial rehabilitation. The control group received traditional vocational services in place at sites. Study was conducted over 24 months, during which employment was tracked weekly and services tracked monthly. *Outcome Measures:* ▪ Labor force information data, including hours worked, earnings, job duties, level of workplace integration ▪ Types and amounts of vocational and clinical services per month ▪ Whether competitive employment was achieved ▪ Working 40 or more hours in a single month ▪ Monthly earnings from paid employment	All 3 employment outcomes were significantly better for the experimental as compared with the comparison group, with the difference increasing over time. 55% of SE participants achieved competitive employment compared with 34% of control group participants. 51% vs. 39% worked 40 or more hours per week. The SE group earned a median of $122/month, compared with $99/month for control group. The results controlled for demographic variables, clinical status, work history, disability status, and study site confounders. These differences between groups increased over the 24-month period.	Participants were not drawn from a national probability sample, which limits generalization to individuals with severe mental illness. Experimental conditions varied across sites; therefore, it would be difficult to re-create the study and grade the quality of the programs. The study did not include a no-treatment group.

			Intervention		
Cook et al. (2005)	Examine the impact of supported employment programs with highly integrated psychiatric and vocational rehabilitation services on vocational outcomes	I—Randomized controlled trial, multisite N = 1,273 8 study sites in Maryland, Connecticut, South Carolina, Pennsylvania, Arizona, Massachusetts, Maine, and Texas were chosen through the Employment Intervention Demonstration Program. Mean age: 38 years; 53% male, 50% White, 30% African American, 14% Hispanic Latino Diagnoses: 51% schizophrenia spectrum, 21% major depression, 16% bipolar	*Intervention* All SE sites included integrated multidisciplinary services 3×/wk to plan employment interventions, placement into competitive employment, development of jobs that matched clients' preferences, immediate job search at clients' pace, and ongoing vocational support. Clinical services included psychiatric evaluation; medication management; individual, family, or couples' counseling; case management; and psychosocial rehabilitation. The control group received traditional vocational services in place at sites. *Outcome Measures:* • Labor force information data, including hours worked, earnings, job duties, and level of workplace integration • Whether competitive employment was achieved • Working 40 or more hours in a single month • Employment Intervention Demonstration Program measure: Types and amounts of vocational and psychiatric services per month. A running cumulative total number of service hours for each of the 2 types of services were calculated monthly for each of the 24 months of the study.	Over the 24-month period, a larger portion (n = 471, 58%) of the participants in the high-integration services programs achieved competitive employment, compared with 21% (n = 98) of participants in the low-integration programs. More than half (n = 431, 53%) of the high-integration participants worked for at least 40 hours in a month, compared with 31% (n = 144) of the low-integration participants. Participants receiving a high number of hours of vocational services were almost 2½ times as likely to work competitively and almost twice as likely to work 40 or more hours in a month.	Participants were not a representative sample of adults with severe mental illness, limiting the generalize ability of the results. The study's measure of service delivery and service volume may have been too simplified for a complex construct. There was redundancy between likelihood of being employed and chances of receiving some type of vocational service. The study did not include a no-treatment group.
Corrigan (1991)	A meta-analysis conducted on studies of adults with psychiatric diagnoses who had received social skills training	I—Meta-analysis Diagnoses: Developmentally disabled and psychotic and nonpsychotic individuals, and legal offenders 73 of 150 empirical articles were included because they reported statistics that could be transformed to effect sizes	*Intervention:* Social skills training content was not specifically described, but included conversation skills, assertiveness training, and problem solving. Techniques included direct instruction, modeling, role play, feedback, homework, and reinforcement. *Outcome Measures:* Brief Psychiatric Rating Scale, Beck Depression Inventory, Social Avoidance and Distress Scale, and Fear of Negative Evaluation Scale were most commonly used to measure acquired skills, symptom reduction and personal adjustment, and maintenance and generalization of effects.	Social skills training strongly and consistently enhanced skill acquisition and maintenance. Outpatient settings facilitated better results than inpatient settings.	Few studies specifically analyzed the content and techniques of the interventions (conversation skills vs. assertiveness, or role play vs. modeling). The meta-analysis covered a wide range of diagnoses.

(continued)

Evidence Table 2. Mental Health—Paid and Unpaid Employment and Education (continued)

Author/Year	Study Objectives	Level/Design/Participants	Intervention and Outcome Measures	Results	Study Limitations
Crowther, Marshall, Bond, & Hurley (2001)	Evaluate the effectiveness of prevocational training and supported employment (SE) in helping individuals with severe mental illness find and obtain competitive employment	I—Systematic review Study included random-ized controlled trials that compared prevocational training with supported employment or standard community care	*Intervention:* 11 trials met inclusion criteria. 5 were prevocational vs. standard (1,204 participants); SE vs. standard care, 1 trial (256 participants); SE vs. prevocational, 5 trials (491 participants). *Measurement Outcomes:* ▪ Number of individuals in competitive employment ▪ Other employment outcomes (form of employment, mean monthly hours worked, mean earnings) were reviewed secondarily	Prevocational vs. standard: 2 studies showed no superior outcome in number in competitive employment. 3 trials showed no superior outcome in any form of em-ployment. SE vs. standard: SE was combined with Assertive Community Treatment (ACT); significant difference supported SE at 24 months in competitive employment and any employment at 12 months. SE vs. prevocational: significant support of SE in competitive employment at 4, 6, 9, 12, 15, and 18 months in all 5 trials. 1 trial showed no significance in any form of employment. 3 trials showed significantly more hours in SE and more monthly earnings.	Cannot generalize to other countries that have different welfare structures. The addition of ACT to a SE group compared with standard care may confound the findings of study in-cluded in the review.
Dilk & Bond (1996)	Evaluate, using meta-analysis, the effective-ness of skills training and the factors that influence effectiveness, such as meth-odological rigor, outcome mea-sures, and ser-vice settings, in individuals with severe mental illness	I—Meta-analysis Articles published between 1970 and 1992, doctoral dissertations, and master's theses Studies with at least 5 participants, Levels I, II, and III 42 of 168 published studies were included; 26 of 41 dissertations/theses were included; 59 between-group and 9 within-group studies were included; 39 studies were randomized controlled trials, 13 had multiple comparison groups, and 39 used a nonstandard-ized treatment protocol	*Intervention:* Training programs taught the following skills: general interpersonal, assertiveness, prevo-cational, ADLs, micro-interpersonal, dating, affective management, and cognitive. Training approaches were either behavioral or cogni-tive–behavioral. Settings included both inpatient and outpatient. *Outcome Measures:* ▪ Skill acquisition ▪ Symptom reduction ▪ Personal adjustment (Global Assessment of Functioning) ▪ Hospitalization ▪ Vocational readiness	Behavior skills training is effective for teaching inpatients interpersonal and assertiveness skills as indicated by measures of skill acquisition and symptom reduction. Duration of training significantly correlates with effect size. Larger effects were noted for situation-specific measures than for skill usage and role functioning.	This study uncovered several patterns that may limit the outcomes noted in the skills train-ing literature, including a paucity of studies examining skills training in settings other than psychiatric hospitals. Because many of the outcome measures were similar to the studied interventions, the authors warned against the generalize ability of the results. Gender and ethnic-ity were not evenly represented. Most skills training studies focused on social skills. The meta-analysis did not reveal a generalization of social functioning to other skill areas, such as role functioning.

Author/Year	Study Objectives	Level/Design/Participants	Intervention and Outcome Measures	Results and Study Limitations
Duncombe (2004)	Determine whether there is a difference between learning the functional living skill of cooking for people with serious and persistent schizophrenia when it is taught in a clinic or in their home	I—Randomized controlled trial $N = 44$ participants with a diagnosis of non-paranoid schizophrenia or schizoaffective; duration of illness at least 5 years. 40.9% (18) women; 59.1% (26) men Mean age: 45.5 years All lived in group homes or supported apartments that had kitchens available. Participants were assigned in 22 pairs matched on cognitive level and randomly assigned to 1 of the 2 groups	*Intervention:* Group 1: Cooking skills training in the home Group 2: Cooking skills training in the clinic Participants received treatment individually 4 times in the designated context with a 1-wk lapse between each session. *Outcome Measures:* Kitchen Task Assessment–Modified (KTA–M)	Both groups posted significant improvement between their pre and post scores on the KTA–M. The results did not show a significant difference in the level of learning between the 2 groups in the different contexts. Qualitative differences in the 2 settings may have affected the results. The clinic was quiet with minimal distractions. The kitchens in the group homes were cluttered and distracting. Multiple intervention sites result in inconsistencies in the research. There may have been a ceiling effect for the KTA–M.
Frank et al. (2008)	Evaluate the effectiveness of interpersonal and social rhythm therapy (IPRST) on occupational functioning for adults with bipolar disorder	I—Randomized controlled trial $N = 175$ participants with a lifetime history of bipolar Type I disorder or schizoaffective disorder, manic type $n = 43$ Intensive Case Management (ICM)/ICM acute/maintenance phase $n = 45$ ICM/IPSRT $n = 48$ IPSRT/ICM $n = 39$ IPSRT/IPSRT	*Intervention:* Participants randomized to groups based on ICM or IPSRT in the acute phase followed by ICM or IPSRT in the maintenance phase. IPSRT stresses the importance of maintaining daily routines and identifying potential rhythm disruptors. ICM a manual-driven approach to the medical management of bipolar disorder that includes education about the disorder, medications, sleep hygiene, and nonspecific support. *Outcome Measures:* UCLA Social Attainment Scale at baseline, end, 1 and 2 years Social Rhythm Metric	Although participants initially assigned to IPRST showed more rapid improvement in occupational functioning as compared to those in ICM, at 2 years there was no difference between groups. The effect was more pronounced for women. Variables that were later found to be associated with outcome, such as marital status and medical burden, were not distributed equally among the maintenance study conditions.

(continued)

Evidence Table 2. Mental Health—Paid and Unpaid Employment and Education (*continued*)

Author/Year	Study Objectives	Level/Design/Participants	Intervention and Outcome Measures	Results	Study Limitations
Gold et al. (2006)	Evaluate the effectiveness of supported employment (SE) programs in a rural setting that differs from an urban setting in that services are more loosely linked and geographically distant and where there may be scarce and less diverse job opportunities.	I—Randomized controlled trial *N* = 143 *n* = 66 in assertive community treatment (ACT)/individual placement and support program (IPS) *n* = 77 in traditional vocational services Participant criteria: Serious mental illness, 18+ years of age, unemployed, current/future interest in employment	*Intervention:* ACT–IPS: Vocational aspects were handled by a team with a staff:participant ratio of 1:10. They searched for jobs of interest and assessed past work, current skills, and tolerance for job demands. Specialists provided unlimited support during study. Control: Case managers, with a staff:participant ratio of 1:30 max. Employment specialists met with the team every 2–4 wk to discuss clients. Both groups' goals were competitive employment. The ACT–IPS group immediately looked for competitive work, but the control group encouraged graduated work-adjustment periods for jobs up to 6 months. *Outcome Measures:* ■ Employment, income earned over time ■ Positive and Negative Syndrome Scale ■ Quality of Life Index	Participants in the ACT–IPS group were significantly more likely to hold competitive jobs than those in the control group (80% vs. 38%). The earnings of the ACT–IPS group also were significantly higher than those of the control group. There was wide variation across both study groups for job tenure. The authors reported that the study outcomes mirror those in urban settings.	The project redesign may have limited internal validity and program construct validity. Possible selection bias and unobserved variables between programs. Neurocognitive status, which could account for competitive work outcomes, was not studied.
Gutman, Kerner, Zombek, Dulek, & Ramsey (2009)	Assess the effectiveness of a supported education (The Bridge Program) program for adults with psychiatric disabilities	I—Randomized controlled trial Follow up to pilot study *N* = 38 participants; *n* = 21 intervention, *n* = 17 control; metropolitan area; 22 men, 16 women; age range: 19–55 Participants recruited from 3 mental health facilities in New York Diagnoses include schizophrenia, schizoaffective disorder, bipolar disorder, depression No participants currently employed. Education levels ranged from not completed high school to completed high school and some college	*Intervention:* The Bridge Program: The program consists of 12 2-hr classroom-lab modules, including time management, stress management, study skills, reading, writing, computer, social skills, and exploration of educational/vocational, followed by 1 hr of mentoring. The program is held 2×/wk for 6 wk. Additional mentoring is offered to participants who complete the program. Faculty and graduate students at Columbia University Occupational Therapy program implemented the program. Control: Treatment as usual at mental health facility. *Outcome Measures:* ■ Program completion rate ■ Educational or job placement rate ■ Measures for program modules ■ Participant Comfort With the Student Role Scale	16 of 21 participants completed The Bridge Program and at 6-month follow-up, 10 of 16 had enrolled in job training, educational program, obtained employment, or were applying for a program. Only 1 of 17 control group participants were involved in coursework. Participants in The Bridge Program showed increased skills in basic academic areas, improved professional behaviors, improved social skills needed for school/work settings. Adherence to a medication routine, having a stable residence, and consistent program attendance were strongest predictors of success in program.	Small sample size; lack of validity and reliability for the pre- and posttests for program modules.

Author/Year	Study Objectives	Level/Design/Participants	Intervention and Outcome Measures	Results	Study Limitations
Hadas-Lidor, Katz, Tyano, & Weizman (2001)	Determine the efficacy of dynamic cognitive treatment, using the Instrumental Enrichment (IE) intervention for clients with schizophrenia in a community day rehabilitation program.	I—Randomized controlled trial $N = 58$ Study group, $n = 29$ Control group, $n = 29$ Participants were diagnosed with schizophrenia in a rehabilitation center in Petah-Tiqva, Israel. The 2 groups were matched for gender, age, family status, education, and category of schizophrenia.	*Intervention:* Study group: 2- to 3-hr sessions for 1 hr of the IE program that combines a remedial and adaptive approach using 15 tools, each focusing on a specific cognitive deficiency, performed by occupational therapists, 1–3 sessions per week. Group treatment every 2–3 wk, voluntary. Control group: Traditional occupational therapy, including functional tasks and expressive activities in groups and individually by occupational therapists, with the same schedule as the study group. All treatments were done at the rehabilitation center. *Outcome Measures:* ■ Learning Potential Assessment Device (memory and thought processes) ■ Raven Progressive Matrices and General Aptitude Test Battery ■ Fitts questionnaire (self-concept) ■ Functional outcomes, IADLs, work and residence status	Participants in the IE study condition performed significantly better on almost all of the cognitive tests as compared with the control group. The IE group also demonstrated significant changes on work and residence status compared with the traditional occupational therapy group. No differences were observed for IADLs and self-concept.	The IADL self-report questionnaire may not have been sensitive enough to detect changes in performance in the schizophrenic population. There was no standardized measure of occupational performance.
Kern, Green, Mintz, & Liberman (2003)	Examine the effectiveness of errorless learning to compensate for neurocognitive deficits in teaching job tasks to adults with schizophrenia and schizoaffective disorder	I—Randomized controlled trial $N = 54$ unemployed, clinically stable adults with schizophrenia or schizoaffective disorder Errorless learning condition, $n = 29$ Conventional trial and error instruction, $n = 25$	*Intervention:* Entry-level job tasks (index card filing and toilet tank assembly) were taught either through errorless learning or trial-and-error learning. *Outcome Measures:* Job task performance—percentage of accuracy scores immediately after training	The errorless learning group scored high in job task performance regardless of neurocognitive impairment. The conventional instruction group showed a close correspondence between job task performance and degree of neurocognitive impairment.	Participants in both conditions were not matched for level of neurocognitive impairment.
Kern, Liberman, Kopelowicz, Mintz, & Green (2002)	Evaluate the effectiveness of errorless learning to teach entry-level job tasks to persons with serious and persistent mental illness	I—Randomized controlled trial $N = 65$ unemployed, clinically stable outpatients with schizophrenia or schizoaffective disorder Errorless learning condition, $n = 32$ Conventional learning condition, $n = 33$	*Intervention:* Entry-level job tasks (index card filing and toilet tank assembly) were taught either through errorless learning or trial-and-error learning in small groups *Outcome Measures:* Accuracy, speed, and overall performance	Although there were significant differences in accuracy for both job tasks, the errorless learning group was superior to the conventional learning group only for the card filing task, and there were no differences for speed of performance. Both groups showed decreases in productivity and accuracy at 3 months.	During the 3-month follow-up period, participants had no exposure to tasks learned, which is different from a real world job situation.

(continued)

Evidence Table 2. Mental Health—Paid and Unpaid Employment and Education (continued)

Author/Year	Study Objectives	Level/Design/Participants	Intervention and Outcome Measures	Results	Study Limitations
Kielhofner & Brinson (1989)	Examine the effectiveness of a theoretically based (model of human occupation) occupational therapy aftercare program for chronic mentally ill persons	I—Randomized controlled trial N = 34 Experimental group, n = 20 Control group, n = 14 Diagnoses: Schizophrenia, schizoaffective disorder, bipolar disorder, major depression, atypical depression, bulimia, anorexia Between the ages of 25–40: 16 female, 18 male	*Intervention:* The aftercare program included 1.5- to 2-hr sessions, 3×/wk for 12 wk. Sessions consisted of small group (6 members) activities led by a therapist. The program comprised a series of goals and strategies derived from the model of human occupation's conceptualization of occupational functioning as a continuum of behaviors from exploration to competence to achievement. Each session was highly structured with specific goals, materials, and equipment listed in the protocol. *Outcome Measures:* Recidivism data; Occupational Questionnaire; Katz Adjustment Scales, and the Level of Performance of Socially Expected Activities Scale measured free time and social activities, volition, work, daily living tasks, and recreation; also, a program evaluation completed from therapist report.	The data supporting the hypotheses were not statistically significant. Data trends indicate a positive impact on recidivism and quality of life. Program evaluation reflects most short-term goals were achieved and many long-term goals were achieved (no comparison with control group). Other results of the program evaluation: ■ Therapist assessed the program to be too short. ■ The highly structured format did not accommodate individual needs. ■ The small groups provided a nonthreatening atmosphere. ■ Positive responses from participants correlated with physical activity.	Small sample size; variability in demographic traits, participation in the program, and outcome variables of subjects; control group was not described; posttest only measured.
Kopelowicz, Wallace, & Zarate (1998)	Examine the effects of brief manualized treatment programs designed to teach patient skills to reenter the community and participate in their own self-care	I—Randomized controlled trial 2 groups randomly assigned to either the community reentry program or occupational therapy. N = 59 adults with schizophrenia or schizoaffective disorder Community reentry group, n = 28 Occupational therapy group, n = 31 Mean age: 35 years	*Intervention:* The community reentry program was provided in a short-stay acute psychiatric inpatient facility. It consisted of 16 training sessions, 45 min long, divided into 2 8-session sections. Training sessions included introducing the program and providing a rationale for learning skills, developing an aftercare treatment plan, and teaching coping skills. A modular skills training approach was used in which 7 learning activities were used to teach each session. 2 trainers from a multidisciplinary staff, including occupational therapy, conducted the sessions. The occupational therapy sessions were described as including a full range of customary occupational therapy activities by 2–3 occupational therapists. *Outcome Measures:* ■ Test of knowledge and performance of material presented. This test consists of 18 questions, problems, and role-playing activities ■ Attendance at aftercare service	Participants in the community reentry group were significantly more likely than those in the occupational therapy group to attend the first aftercare appointment. The scores from the test of knowledge and performance for the community reentry group increased from 55% correct preintervention to 81% correct postintervention. For the occupational therapy group, the increase did not change significantly (50%–55%). There was a significant difference between the 2 groups.	Participants were followed for only 1 month after discharge. The outcome measures were designed to measure the specific items taught in the community reentry program. It is not clear whether the occupational therapy groups were working on the same objectives.

Citation	Study Objectives	Level/Design	Intervention and Outcome Measures	Results	Limitations/Notes
Latimer et al. (2006)	Determine the effectiveness of the individual placement and support model and compare outcomes with a nonsupported employment vocational program in Canada	I—Randomized controlled trial N = 150 participants Supported employment (SE) group, n = 75 Traditional vocational services group, n = 75 Inclusion criteria: 18–64 years; diagnosis of schizophrenia, bipolar disorder, or major depression; unemployed	*Intervention:* SE group: Participants were assigned to an employment specialist who helped them define a competitive job according to interest, obtain a job, continue in a job, recover from job loss, and continue in new search and investigate problems. Participants also had a case manager and psychiatrist. Traditional vocational services group: Chose services from the following: sheltered workshop, creative workshop, client programs. Job skills and psychosocial groups were also available. *Outcome Measures:* ■ Clients were interviewed every 2 months to record job start and end dates, hr/wk, salary, and type of work. ■ Quality of life, social network, self-esteem ■ Psychiatric symptoms	The SE group had higher employment rates (any paid or competitive) in each of the 12 months, with significant differences in competitive work. There were no differences between groups for total hours worked and wages earned.	This program was done in Canada, a country that allows more monthly earnings with disability income than in the United States. The percentage of participants who spent time in competitive employment in any given month was no more than 27%, which is lower than similar studies in the past. The authors suggested that institutional environments and implementation issues could account for the differences. The study was started at the same time as the SE program. A study done after the program has been used for a longer time may result in different outcomes.
Lee, Tan, Ma, Tsai, & Liu (2006)	Examine the effect of a work-related stress management program on perceived work-related stress in patients with chronic schizophrenia	I—Randomized controlled trial N = 29 patients with schizophrenia in a psychiatric hospital who were employed part-time in the hospital's job program center. Group A: 12 men, 2 women; mean age: 41.21 years Group B: 10 men, 5 women; mean age: 37.53 years	*Intervention:* Crossover design: Group A received treatment for 12 wk, then no treatment for 12 wk. Group B did the opposite. A work-stress management group was held 1× /wk for 1 hr in the occupational therapy department in the psychiatric center. The group addressed the effects of stress on cognition, behavior, and emotion to help them monitor their stressors and symptoms. Skills training, assertiveness training, and problem-solving skills training also were addressed. *Outcome Measures:* Work-related stress questionnaire for chronic psychiatric patients	Participants' stress levels significantly decreased during the stress management program. These increases were not maintained in the following 12 wk when the stress management program was not taking place.	Some situations described in the outcome measure were not encountered by participants, and therefore the stress scores would be lower. The program was not designed for individuals with lower cognitive levels. The study examined only the in-house employment program.

(continued)

Evidence Table 2. Mental Health—Paid and Unpaid Employment and Education (continued)

Author/Year	Study Objectives	Level/Design/Participants	Intervention and Outcome Measures	Results	Study Limitations
Liberman et al. (1998)	Compare the effect of a manualized social skills training program with a crafts- and task-based occupational therapy intervention conducted by trained paraprofessionals on community functioning of persons with persistent forms of schizophrenia	I—Randomized controlled trial *N* = 84, randomized within cohorts of 10–12 patients, 100% male, 66% White, 25% African American, 9% Hispanic or Asian; diagnosis of schizophrenia	*Intervention:* Group 1 received psychosocial occupational therapy in which participants' interests and abilities were individualized through arts and crafts, discussion of feelings, and articulation of personal goals. Three occupational therapists provided services 4 days/wk for 3 hr/day. Group 2 received skills training conducted by 1 occupational therapist and 3 paraprofessionals using the UCLA Social and Independent Living Skills Program, a manualized education protocol covering basic conversation, recreation for leisure, medication management, and symptom management. Training occurred 4 days/wk for 3 hr/day. *Outcome Measures:* • Independent Living Skills Survey • Social Activities Scale • Profile of Adaptation to Life • Rosenberg Self-Esteem Scale • Brief Symptom Inventory • Lehman Quality of Life Scale	Participants in the intervention group showed significant improvement on independent living skills, significant improvement from pretreatment to posttreatment on the Rosenberg Self-Esteem Scale and Brief Symptom Inventory, and significant improvement for the skills trained group on Distress Factor I of the Profile of Adaptation to Life. Both groups showed significant pretreatment-to-posttreatment improvement on the Social Activities Scale, the Global Assessment Scale, and the Brief Psychiatric Rating Scale.	Case managers were not blinded to the treatment conditions.
McGurk, Mueser, Feldman, Wolfe, & Pascaris (2007)	Evaluate the effectiveness of a cognitive training program for schizophrenia, the Thinking Skills for Work Program that was integrated into supported employment services	I—Randomized controlled trial *N* = 44 persons with severe mental illness at 2 sites Intervention, *n* = 23 Control, *n* = 21	*Intervention:* Supported employment plus the Thinking Skills for Work program that provides computerized cognitive training program. Control: Supported Employment alone *Outcome Measures:* Measures of competitive employment—total number of jobs, total wages, total number of hours and weeks worked	Following a 2- to 3-year follow-up period, those in the Thinking Skills for Work and supported employment were more likely to work, held more jobs, worked more weeks, worked more hours, and earned more wages than participants in the supported employment alone condition.	Sites varied with respect to fidelity to the supported employment model; small group size; lack of follow-up of cognitive measures

Citation	Study Objectives	Level/Design/Participants	Intervention and Outcome Measures	Results	Study Limitations
McGurk, Twamley, Sitzer, McHugo, & Mueser (2007)	Evaluate the effects of cognitive remediation for improving cognitive performance, symptoms, and psychosocial functioning in schizophrenia	I—Meta-analysis 26 randomized controlled trials with 1,151 patients with schizophrenia, schizophreniform disorder, or schizoaffective disorder	*Intervention:* The studies included examined psychosocial interventions designed to improve cognitive performance. *Outcome Measures:* The meta-analysis included studies with at least 1 neuropsychological measure that examined generalization of effects rather than assessment on trained tasks only.	The results indicate that there were significant improvements for all outcomes. There were medium effect sizes for cognitive performance and psychosocial functioning and a small effect size for symptoms. The effects of cognitive remediation on psychosocial functioning were stronger for those studies that paired cognitive remediation with psychiatric rehabilitation rather than in those that examined cognitive remediation alone.	Study is of good quality.
Mueser et al. (2005)	Evaluate the effectiveness of supplementary social skills training on improving work outcomes for clients enrolled in supported employment programs	I—Randomized controlled trial $N = 35$ Group 1, $n = 18$ Group 2, $n = 17$ All clients were enrolled in supported employment or employed at a job obtained in the last 2 months Mean age: 37.7 years Diagnoses: Schizophrenia or schizoaffective disorder, major depression or bipolar disorder, other psychiatric diagnoses	*Intervention:* Group 1: Supported employment (control group) includes rapid job search, individualized job matches, individualized and time-unlimited follow-along supports. 2 hrs of support/wk avg. Group 2: Supported employment plus workplace fundamentals program, a manualized intervention designed to teach clients skills for succeeding in the workplace. Skill areas addressed include making work changes, learning about workplace stressors, problem solving, managing mental and physical health, improving job performance. Sessions were 2 hrs, 1×/wk. Approx. 3–4 months to complete program; monthly booster sessions were offered. *Outcome measures:* ■ Vocational outcomes: hours worked, wages earned, and supported employment services utilized were tracked weekly ■ Workplace Fundamentals Knowledge Test	The workplace fundamentals group showed significantly more improvement in their workplace knowledge than the control group. There was a trend for more clients in the workplace fundamentals group to be working during the 18-month follow-up, but it was not statistically significant. The groups did not differ in number of hours worked or wages earned.	The clients in this study had higher levels of education and longer job tenure histories than clients typically enrolled in supported employment services, so the results may differ with clients that may be more in need of supplementary skills training. Small sample resulted in low power to detect effects of the workplace fundamentals program on employment outcomes. Information on job satisfaction was not obtained; job satisfaction is a goal of the workplace fundamentals program. Symptoms and quality of life ratings were not obtained.

(continued)

Evidence Table 2. Mental Health—Paid and Unpaid Employment and Education *(continued)*

Author/Year	Study Objectives	Level/Design/Participants	Intervention and Outcome Measures	Results	Study Limitations
Mueser et al. (2004)	Compare the work outcomes of 3 vocational rehabilitation models for persons with severe mental illness: (1) the individual placement and support (IPS), (2) a psychosocial rehabilitation (PSR) program using transitional employment, and (3) standard vocational services. This study also examined social outcomes of these models.	I—Randomized controlled trial $N = 204$ IPS group, $n = 68$ PSR group, $n = 67$ Standard services group, $n = 69$ Participants were clients with mental illness receiving services at a community mental health center.	*Intervention:* IPS model: Employment specialists served on a client's psychiatric treatment team to integrate services. The employment specialist provided a range of services, including engagement of services, exploring job interests, obtaining a job, and job support. Outreach was based on the assertive community treatment model, with an emphasis on services being delivered in the client's natural setting. PSR model: Clients participated in a series of preparatory training activities, followed by transitional jobs, followed by assistance with obtaining competitive work. The program was located off-site from the mental health center. Standard services group: Involved an array of vocational programs offered off-site from the mental health center. Comprehensive employment data were collected for 2 years, and interviews were conducted at baseline and every 6 months for 2 years thereafter. *Outcome Measures:* ▪ Structured Clinical Interview for *DSM–IV* for diagnostic and background information ▪ Employment outcomes (interview and Indiana Job Satisfaction Scale) ▪ Nonvocational outcomes (Positive and Negative Syndrome Scale, Global Assessment Scale, Social Adjustment Scale II, modified Social Support and Social Network Interview, Brief Version of the Quality of Life Interview, Alcohol Use Scale, and Drug Use Scale)	For competitive work, post hoc pairwise comparisons indicated significantly better IPS outcomes than PSR or standard services, which did not differ. For all paid employment, IPS clients had better outcomes than PSR and standard services clients, and standard services clients had better outcomes than PSR clients. Job satisfaction did not differ among groups. Retention rates over 2 years remained over 90% for IPS clients, compared with 50%–60% for PSR clients and <40% for standard services clients. There were few differences between the programs on nonvocational outcomes. Only 2 effects were significant: Global Assessment Scale scores tended to improve over time, and cognitive function tended to worsen over time for all groups. There was a trend for clients in the PSR group to show more satisfaction with their social relationships over time.	The IPS and PSR programs had Spanish-speaking vocational staff; standard services did not. Interviewers were not blind to vocational program assignment. The PSR program was not an International Center for Clubhouse Development–certified clubhouse; therefore, results cannot be generalized to clubhouse programs.
Patterson et al. (2003)	Evaluate the efficacy of a skills training program to improve functioning in middle-age and older adults with chronic psychotic disorders	I—Randomized controlled trial $N = 40$ patients at a board-and-care facility Intervention group, $n = 16$ Control group, $n = 16$ (8 dropouts)	*Intervention:* Intervention group received 24-session Functional Adaptation Skills Training (FAST), a manualized social–cognitive theory–based behavioral intervention focused on improving medication management, social skills, communication skills, organization and planning, transportation, and financial management. Control group received treatment as usual. *Outcome Measures:* ▪ UCSD Performance-Based Skills Assessment (functional skills) ▪ Positive and Negative Syndromes Scales ▪ Hamilton Rating Scale for Depression ▪ Quality of Well-Being Scale	Functional performance following participation in the FAST program improved significantly postintervention and was maintained at 3-month follow-up in comparison to control participants. There was no change in psychopathology during the treatment and follow-up periods.	Performance-based functional measure may not accurately portray real-life performance. Client contact was greater for the FAST condition than for the control condition, which may explain differences in results.

Patterson et al. (2005)	Evaluate the effectiveness of the Program for Training and Development of Skills in Latinos (PEDAL) on improving everyday functioning compared with a time-equivalent friendly support group	I—Randomized controlled trial Participants were selected from three mental health clinics near the U.S.–Mexico border in San Diego County. 100% of participants were Latino, of Mexican descent, and Spanish-speaking $N = 29$ participants Group 1, $n = 21$ (mean age: 46.8 years) Group 2, $n = 8$ (mean age: 57.3 years) Diagnoses: Schizophrenia or schizoaffective disorder	*Intervention:* Group 1 (PEDAL) received a manualized, cognitive-behavioral intervention that focuses on 6 areas of everyday functioning (medication management, social skills, communication skills, organization and planning, transportation, and financial management). PEDAL is an adapted for the Latino population from an existing program, Functional Adaptation Skills Training. Group 2 (control) took part in a time-equivalent, friendly support group that focused on a current theme being discussed and encouraged problem solving. Specific skills were not taught. *Outcome Measures:* ■ Social Skills Performance Assessment (SSPA) ■ USCD Performance-Based Skills Assessment ■ Role-playing tasks involving social and communication skills, household management, and general organization	Group 1 showed significant improvement over Group 2 in everyday functioning at 6 months. Group 1 showed improvements in everyday functioning at 12 and 18 months, but the effect size was not significant. There was no difference between groups for performance on the Social Skills Performance Assessment.	Small sample size. Performance-based assessments were conducted in laboratory settings. Gender, patterns of symptoms, past history, family involvement, and the importance of specific cultural factors were not examined. Findings may not generalize beyond Latinos of Mexican descent.
Patterson et al. (2006)	Evaluate the effectiveness of Functional Adaptation Skills Training (FAST) on improving functional and social skills on outpatients with chronic psychotic disorders	I—Randomized controlled trial $N = 240$ FAST group, $n = 124$ Control group, $n = 116$ Participants were recruited from 25 board-and-care facilities in San Diego County and then randomly assigned to groups. Diagnosis: Schizophrenia or schizoaffective disorder	*Intervention:* Participants for both groups met 1×/wk for 24 wk for 120 min/session. Group 1 (FAST) received a manualized behavioral intervention targeting 6 areas of everyday functioning (medication management, social skills, communication skills, organization and planning, transportation, and financial management). Groups were co-led by a graduate-level therapist and a management or nursing paraprofessional. Group 2 (attention control condition) received support intervention sessions that addressed personal problems and what themes emerged; solutions were not discussed. *Outcome Measures:* ■ UCSD Performance-Based Skills Assessment ■ Social skills performance assessment ■ Medication management abilities assessment ■ Positive and Negative Syndromes Scale (PANNS) ■ Hamilton Rating Scale for Depression (HAM–D) ■ Quality of Well-Being Scale	FAST participants improved more on everyday living skills and social skills than the control group. There was no difference between groups for medication management. Groups did not differ in overall improvement of secondary outcomes such as HAM–D and PANSS scores.	Exclusion of the participant's support network. Results of participants recruited from board-and-care facilities may not generalize to other settings.

(continued)

Evidence Table 2. Mental Health—Paid and Unpaid Employment and Education (continued)

Author/Year	Study Objectives	Level/Design/Participants	Intervention and Outcome Measures	Results	Study Limitations
Pilling et al. (2002)	Provide a meta-analytical review of social skills training and cognitive remediation in treating persons with schizophrenia	I—Meta-analysis of randomized controlled trials 9 social skills studies; studies based on samples of people with schizophrenia or related disorders, including delusional disorder, schizophreniform disorder, and schizoaffective disorder	*Intervention:* Structured psychosocial interventions (group or individual) intended to enhance social performance and reduce distress and difficulty in social situations. *Outcome Measures:* ■ Brief Psychiatric Rating Scale ■ Global Adjustment Scale ■ Social skills changes ■ Relapse ■ Medication compliance ■ Quality of life, adaptation of life, social adjustment ■ Harm to others, harm to self	Overall, the meta-analyses did not reveal a difference between social skills and comparison treatments.	The studies varied significantly in the outcome measures.
Robertson, Connaughton, & Nicol (1998)	Determine the effectiveness of life skills training programs vs. standard care for individuals with chronic mental illness	I—Meta-analysis Included randomized controlled trials and quasi-randomized controlled trials, 129 citations reviewed—2 studies included	*Intervention:* Group or individual training programs involving independent functioning in daily living. Examples include money management, home management, domestic skills, and personal self-care. Social skills training was not a focus. Comparison groups were considered traditional rehabilitation, including recreation, art, and occupational therapy. *Outcome Measures:* ■ Life skills, social functioning ■ Behavior ■ Economic outcomes ■ Social Anxiety Scale ■ Royal Edinburgh Occupational Therapy Assessment Form	The results were inconclusive, providing no evidence for or against life skills training programs.	The sample size in the studies included was too small to draw any firm conclusions, possibly indicating that the selection criteria were too restrictive.

| Rogers, Anthony, Lyass, & Penk (2006) | Examine and compare the effectiveness of psychiatric vocational rehabilitation (PVR) and enhanced state vocational rehabilitation (ESVR) in improving employment, educational, clinical, and quality of life outcomes for persons with psychiatric disabilities | I—Randomized controlled trial

N = 135
PVR group, n = 70
ESVR group, n = 65

Participants had a major mental illness, were unemployed or substantially underemployed, and expressed a desire for vocational rehabilitation services | Intervention:
The PVR group intervention was based on the Choose–Get–Keep model that outlines how practitioners diagnose, plan, and intervene to help persons with psychiatric disabilities develop skills to be successful and satisfied in employment. It included classroom instruction and individual meetings for 24 months.

ESVR participants were referred for state vocational rehabilitation services, including counseling, guidance, referral, training, and treatment as appropriate. The duration varied according to their individual rehabilitation plans.

Outcome Measures:
Major assessments were conducted at baseline, 9 months, 18 months, and 24 months postbaseline.
■ Rosenberg Self-Esteem Scale
■ Change Assessment Scale
■ Brief Psychiatric Rating Scale
■ Lehman Quality of Life Interview
■ Vocational/educational status instruments | Both measures were deemed effective by the authors.
There was no significant difference in the vocational, self-esteem, quality of life, or symptomatology outcomes of the individuals who received the PVR intervention vs. those who received ESVR. | The authors took substantial measures to discourage ESVR participants from dropping out. This may have contaminated the study results. |
| Torres, Mendez, Merino, & Moran (2002) | Examine the effectiveness of using El Tren, a board game, to improve social functioning for persons with schizophrenia | I—Randomized controlled trial

N = 49 Spanish-speaking clients participating in the hospital's day rehabilitation center
Group 1, n = 19
Group 2, n = 16
Group 3, n = 14
36 male, 13 female

Most were single, living with immediate family in an urban area, and unemployed | Intervention:
Group 1 played El Tren, a board game that simulates a railway trip in which unexpected problems are encountered and solved as the train passes through each station; received social skills training that focused on teaching clients to receive, process, and send social communication signals; received psychomotor skills training, which included exercise to develop equilibrium, rhythm, and coordination; and took part in occupational therapy, with activities designed to improve fine and gross motor movements.
Group 2 received social skills training, psychomotor skills training, and occupational therapy but did not play El Tren.
Group 3's program included occupational therapy only.

Frequency:
■ El Tren 1 hr/wk
■ Social skills training 3 hr/wk
■ Occupational therapy: 5 hr/wk
Duration: 6 months

Outcome Measures:
Social Function Scale | Participants in Group 1 achieved significant improvement in social withdrawal, interpersonal functioning, recreational activities, and work over time.
Participants in Group 2 achieved significant improvement in social withdrawal, independence (performance), and work.
Participants in Group 3 showed significant improvements in social activities and work.
Participants in Group 1 had significantly more improvement in interpersonal functioning than those in the other groups. There also was significantly more improvement in Group 1 than Group 2 on social withdrawal but not for Group 3. | El Tren has been tested at only 1 center.
The results may not generalize to other populations. |

Evidence Table 2. Mental Health—Paid and Unpaid Employment and Education (continued)

Author/Year	Study Objectives	Level/Design/Participants	Intervention and Outcome Measures	Results	Study Limitations
Tsang, Chan, Wong, & Liberman (2009)	Evaluate the effectiveness of an integrated supported employment (ISE) program that combines Individual Placement and Support (IPS) with social skills training (SST) for persons with persistent and severe mental illness in Hong Kong	I—Randomized controlled trial $N = 163$ $n = 52$ ISE $n = 56$ IPS $n = 55$ traditional vocational rehabilitation (TVR)	*Intervention:* Group 1: ISE combines IPS with SST, a program to improve social communication, social problem-solving, and social functioning. The IPS program includes referral, building a relationship, vocational assessment, individual employment plan, obtaining employment, and follow-along support. SST is initiated during vocational assessment. Group 2: ISE alone. ISE and IPS groups conducted by occupational therapists Group 3: TVR included comprehensive vocational assessment and prevocational training. *Outcome Measures:* ■ Employment rate ■ Job characteristics ■ Job tenure ■ Salary	After 15 months of participation in services, the ISE participants had significantly higher employment rates and longer job tenure than those in IPS and TVR. Those in IPS had better employment outcomes than those in TVR.	Fidelity to SST and improvement on social skills was not evaluated. Follow-up period may not have been long enough to detect non-vocational and long-term vocational outcomes.
Tsang & Pearson (2001)	Evaluate the effectiveness of a work-related social skills training program in improving the ability to find and keep jobs for persons with schizophrenia	I—Randomized controlled trial $N = 97$ participants recruited from halfway houses and sheltered workshops in Hong Kong Group 1, $n = 30$ Group 2, $n = 26$ Group 3, $n = 41$ All unemployed. Education of no fewer than 5 years of primary school and no more than 5 years of secondary school. Individuals with learning disabilities were excluded. Diagnosis: schizophrenia	*Intervention:* Work-related social skills training program; sessions reviewed basic social skills (e.g., facial expressions/gestures) and social survival skills (personal appearance) and then focused on skills related to finding and keeping a job, conflict resolution, and problem-solving skills. Group 1 received work-related social skills training plus follow-up contact with group members and the trainer. Group 2 received work-related social skills training with no follow-up. Group 3 (comparison group) received standard outpatient psychiatric care. *Outcome Measures:* ■ 2-part measure of work related social competence that evaluated perceived social competence and assessed job-related social performance through role play ■ Motivation questionnaire ■ Employment status	Groups 1 and 2 scored significantly higher on most items, excluding "instructing a new colleague." Groups 1 and 2 scored significantly higher on the role-play test. At the 3-month follow-up assessment, 46.7% of Group 1 was gainfully employed, 23.1% of Group 2 was gainfully employed, and 2.4% of Group 3 was gainfully employed. The differences among groups were statistically significant.	A yearlong follow-up would have been a better predictor of job retention. The study was carried out during a labor shortage in Hong Kong, so jobs were more readily available.

Author (Year)	Purpose	Design/Sample	Intervention/Outcome Measures	Results	Limitations
Twamley, Jeste, & Lehman (2003)	Examine, using a meta-analysis of randomized controlled trials (RCTs), the effectiveness of work rehabilitation interventions for persons with schizophrenia and other primary psychotic disorders	I—Meta-analysis Databases searched: MEDLINE (1966–2002), PsycINFO (1887–2002) Criteria included English-language, peer-reviewed RCTs, reference lists of identified articles 11 studies included for a total of 1,617 participants. Mean sample size: 147 Mean age: 38 years 58% male	*Intervention:* Work rehabilitation approaches from 3 categories: (1) supported employment (SE) or Individual Placement and Support Model (IPS); (2) job-related social skills training; and (3) Incentive Therapy—a Veterans Affairs–based program that offers part-time, set-aside job placements at the VA hospital, compensated at rates below minimum wage. Interventions were provided in an outpatient setting. Control conditions included treatment-as-usual, psychosocial vocational rehabilitation programs, and interventions that differed from the experimental condition by a single variable (e.g., paid vs. unpaid). *Outcome Measures:* ■ Percentages of participants achieving employment ■ Number of hours worked ■ Mean ages earned ■ Mean job tenure	9 of the 11 studies reported positive results for IPS/SE programs. Mean effect size comparing IPS/SE to conventional vocational rehabilitation = 0.79; however, nearly half (49%) did not obtain competitive work. The single Incentive Therapy study and the single work-related social skills training article found improved participation in working at end point. Across all RCTs, the weighted mean effect size for employment in the experimental vs. comparison conditions was 0.66.	The number of RCTs of vocational rehabilitation restricted to individuals with schizophrenia is limited. The number of RCTs of work rehabilitation approaches other than IPS/SE is very limited.
Velligan et al. (2000)	Evaluate the effectiveness of cognitive adaptation training on levels of adaptive functioning in outpatients with schizophrenia	I—Randomized controlled trial *N* = 45 adults with schizophrenia or schizoaffective disorder post discharge from inpatient psychiatric facility. 15 per group Age range: 18–55 years; Mean age: 37.12 years	*Intervention:* Cognitive adaptation training is a manual-driven series of compensatory strategies based on neuropsychological, behavioral, and occupational therapy principles. An environmental assessment identified triggers for maladaptive behaviors, presence of safety hazards, availability of needed equipment and supplies, and organization of belongings. The person's environment is adapted based on behavior and executive functioning. The groups were seen weekly for a 9-month period. Standard medication follow-up group Control group: Group controlling for therapist contact times and or changes in the patient's environment plus standard follow-up *Outcome Measures:* Brief Psychiatric Rating Scale, Negative Symptom Assessment, Global Assessment of Functioning Scale, Multnomah Community Ability Scale and Relapse	Patients who received cognitive adaptation training did better than those in the control and follow-up–only conditions with respect to level of symptoms and level of adaptive functioning. Relapse rates also improved for this group. Patients in the control condition that included a therapist's weekly home visit and manipulation of the environment in nonspecific ways fared worse than the follow-up–only group.	Small sample size. Lack of a therapeutically active control condition. It is not known if the results would apply to more stable outpatients.

(continued)

Evidence Table 2. Mental Health—Paid and Unpaid Employment and Education (continued)

Author/Year	Study Objectives	Level/Design/Participants	Intervention and Outcome Measures	Results	Study Limitations
Velligan et al. (2006)	Examine the usage rates of environmental supports provided through cognitive adaptation training vs. a generic environmental supports group	I—Randomized controlled trial $N = 68$, but 3-month data available only for 60 Group 1, $n = 29$ Group 2, $n = 31$ Outpatients with schizophrenia or schizoaffective disorder receiving 2nd-generation antipsychotic medication other than clozapine	*Intervention:* Group 1: Cognitive adaptation training: a manual-driven series of environment supports—such as signs, checklists, supplies—that are individually tailored, set up in the home environment, and reinforced weekly. Group 2: Generic environmental supports: a manual-driven series of generic supports (e.g., calendars, pill containers, alarm clocks) are given to clients in the clinic. Clients are expected to set up supports on their own using an audio recording of the trainers and clients "how-to" discussion. Group 3: Assessment only Frequency/duration Group 1: 30 min/wk Group 2: 1 visit for initial training (time not reported), follow-up phone calls 1 time/month *Outcome Measures:* Each month a utilization researcher telephoned each client and asked about frequency of use of the item and how the item was used	Participants in Group 1 reported significantly higher use rates of environmental supports than Group 2.	Utilization researchers were not blinded to which treatment group the participant belonged. It is unclear whether the higher rate use of Group 1 was due the individualization of supports, the training in the use of the supports, or the weekly visits that reinforce use of the supports. May not generalize to other groups with severe mental illnesses.
Level II					
Bell & Bryson (2003)	Predict the rate of improvement over time on measures of work performance using the Work Behavior Inventory (WBI) and neuropsychological battery scores	II—Cohort study $N = 33$ participants diagnosed with schizophrenia or schizoaffective disorder who had completed 22–26 wk of work rehabilitation. 6 participants dropped out of a no-pay group.	*Intervention:* Participants were placed in 26-wk work placements from 20 work sites. Work performance was evaluated biweekly (total: 13) by the WBI. The information was analyzed to separate the participants into those who had improved WBI scores (20% or more) and those who did not. The subscales of the WBI were analyzed within each biweekly evaluation. The slopes of improvement were analyzed with other evaluations to predict the WBI slopes. *Outcome Measures:* ■ Wisconsin Card Sorting Test, Wechsler Adult Intelligence Scale, Continuous Performance Test, Wechsler Memory Scale–Revised, Hopkins Verbal Learning Test, Gorham Proverbs Test, and the Bell–Lysaker Emotion Recognition Test were all used to measure cognitive, emotional and intelligence levels. ■ The WBI was used for work factors.	Participants either achieved proficiency or improved their performance on the 5 domains of the WBI by 76%–91% over the 26 wk of participation in the work program. Individual differences on the cognitive tests predicted rates of improvement on the WBI.	Study was done only with men in their late 40s with an extended history of mental disorder. The results did not look at the superior performance of individuals from start to finish or those who did not improve above 29%. Results would likely differ in those groups. Results may differ over extended study period.

Reference	Purpose	Design/Sample	Intervention/Outcome Measures	Results	Limitations
Kates, Nikolaou, Ballie, & Hess (1997)	Evaluate the effectiveness of an in-home employment program for persons with severe mental illness	II—Nonrandomized control N = 52 n = 26 individuals with a mental illness who did not have access to work programs n = 26 (control group) Individuals cross-matched on age, sex, diagnosis, and number of hospital admissions. Diagnoses: Schizophrenia, affective psychosis	*Intervention:* In-home program: A specific work project would be decided on by staff and client. The components for the work tasks were brought to the client's home, where clients would complete the work in their own time. The staff would visit twice a week to measure progress, collect work, replace tasks, or pay the client. Control program: Outpatient program of sponsoring mental health program *Outcome Measures:* ■ Beck Depression Scale ■ Rosenberg Self-Esteem Questionnaire ■ 90-item symptom checklist ■ General Health Questionnaire ■ Information on earnings, productivity and work outcomes, hospitalization rates, cost analysis	Although there was no difference in symptoms at 12 months, there was a significant difference between groups at 24 months. Significant improvements in the in-home group were noted at 12 and 24 months. There were no differences between groups on the Beck Depression Scale or the General Health Questionnaire. 5 members of the in-home group joined another work program at the end of this program, as compared with 2 members of the control group. 7 of the in-home group joined the clinical work group. The in-home participants worked an average of 26 hours each month, and their earnings were 3 times that of individuals at local sheltered workshops.	The program consisted of a small group of individuals; lack of randomization.
O'Carroll, Russell, Lawrie, & Johnstone (1999)	Compare the effectiveness of errorless learning over trial-and-error learning	II—Nonrandomized controlled trial N = 61 adults n = 20 adults with memory impairment and schizophrenia n = 21 adults with schizophrenia but no memory impairment n = 20 healthy controls	*Intervention:* All groups received trials with errorless learning and trial-and-error learning. *Outcome Measures:* ■ Mini Mental State Examination ■ Krawiecka Psychiatric Assessment Scale ■ Level of interest/cooperation during test	Although participants with memory impairment had decreased performance on trial-and-error learning compared with the other groups, there was no difference between groups on errorless learning.	Lack of randomization assignment to treatment conditions.

(continued)

Evidence Table 2. Mental Health—Paid and Unpaid Employment and Education (continued)

Author/Year	Study Objectives	Level/Design/Participants	Intervention and Outcome Measures	Results	Study Limitations

Razzano et al. (2005)	Examine the relationship of client clinical factors to employment outcomes	II—Cohort design
		
		$N = 1,273$
		Male: 53%
		Female: 47%
		
		Setting: 8 settings in Maryland, Connecticut, South Carolina, Arizona, Massachusetts, Maine, and Texas
			Intervention:
			Participants completed the 24-month Employment Intervention Demonstration Program (EIDP), $N = 1,273$ a multisite of supported employment intervention
			
			Outcome Measures:
			■ Positive and Negative Syndrome Scales (PANSS)
			■ Alcohol Use Scale and Drug Use Scale
			■ Adherence to medication
			■ Hospitalization
			■ Labor force information data, including hours worked, earnings, job duties, level of workplace integration
			  ■ Types and amounts of vocational and clinical services per month
			  ■ Whether competitive employment was achieved
			  ■ Working 40 or more hours in a single month
			  ■ Monthly earnings from paid employment
				With each month of the study, participants' likelihood of achieving competitive employment increased by approximately 20%.
				
				Higher-than-median PANSS scores on positive symptoms were associated with greater likelihood of achieving competitive employment, whereas higher-than-median negative symptoms were associated with a lesser likelihood of achieving competitive employment.
					EIDP participants were selected from specific sites in certain regions of the United States rather than drawn from a national probability sample of individuals with psychiatric disabilities.

Schindler (2005)	Examine whether adults diagnosed with schizophrenia demonstrated improved task, interpersonal skills, and social roles when involved in a individualized intervention based on the Role Development Program (RDP), in comparison to an intervention based on a multidepartmental activity program (MAP)	II—Nonrandomized controlled trial I = 84 participants, 42 per group, all male Diagnosis: schizophrenia disorder	*Intervention:* Group 1 (comparison): MAP—a non-individualized, therapeutic intervention designed to encourage the productive use of time and socialization in a group setting. Does not address social roles or skills imbedded in social roles. Group 2 (experimental): RDP—an enhancement of the MAP. Utilizes individualized theory-based interventions to help each participant develop task and interpersonal skills within meaningful social roles. Frequency: Both groups received 15 min/wk of individual attention. Other meeting times are not reported. Duration: Varied from 4, 8, and 12 wk *Outcome Measures:* ■ Role Functioning Scale ■ Task Skills Scale ■ Interpersonal Skills Scale	Participants in the RDP demonstrated greater improvement in social roles, task skills, and interpersonal skills than participants in the MAP.	Results may not generalize to individuals in other treatment settings. Staff involved in the RDP may not be typical of staff in other treatment settings. Full validity studies had not been conducted on 2 of the assessment instruments.

Author/Year	Study Objectives	Level/Design/Participants	Intervention and Outcome Measures	Results	Study Limitations
Twamley et al. (2005)	Examine employment outcomes among middle-aged and older clients with schizophrenia in 3 work rehabilitation programs that vary in emphasis	II—Nonrandomized trial, combination of Level III data with randomized controlled trial data $N = 66$ Group 1, $n = 36$ Group 2 $n = 14$ Group 3, $n = 16$	*Intervention:* Group 1 took part in Wellness and Vocational Enrichment (WAVE), which provided prevocational counseling and employment. Participants work 20 hr/wk. Duration varied. All participants had been given the opportunity to receive services for at least 5 months. Group 2 received services from the Department of Rehabilitation/Employment Services (DOR), providing evaluation, job preparation, development and retention services for 12 months. Group 3 received Individual Placement Support (IPS), which provides assessment, support for job searching, and employment support for 12 months. *Outcome Measures:* Participation in work of volunteer activities	81% of IPS participants obtained volunteer or paid work, compared with 44% of WAVE participants and 29% of DOR participants. Rates of competitive work were 69% for IPS, 29% for DOR, and 17% for WAVE. IPS participants were more likely to work than WAVE or DOR participants, suggesting that the place-then-train approach is more effective.	The numbers of participants in the IPS and DOR groups were small. The data from the WAVE group were gathered retrospectively. The IPS and DOR groups received treatment at a university-based mental health clinic, and the WAVE participants received treatment at a VA community mental health clinic.
Level III					
Brown, Rempfer, & Hamer (2002)	Identify strategies that support the acquisition of skills for independent living by examining a program designed to establish habit patterns related to grocery shopping skills.	III—Pretest/posttest $N = 38$ participants Mean age: 40.2 years Diagnoses of schizophrenia or schizoaffective disorder	*Intervention:* 9 sessions included multiple strategies from a variety of learning theories used to teach grocery shopping skills. These strategies included repeated practice with feedback, motivational incentives, scripting of the process, situated cognition approaches, and cuing. *Outcome Measures:* Test of Grocery Shopping Skills—measures accuracy, redundancy, and time to find 10 items in an actual grocery store.	Participants showed statistically significant improvement in accuracy and redundancy of grocery shopping skills but not in time.	No control group for comparison. Limited information available on the demographics. Specific details of the intervention were not provided limiting replication of the study.

(continued)

Author/Year	Study Objectives	Level/Design/Participants	Intervention and Outcome Measures	Results	Study Limitations
Gutman et al. (2007)	Assess the effectiveness of a supported education (The Bridge Program) program for adults with psychiatric disabilities.	III—Pretest/posttest N = 18 participants with a diagnosis of meital illness currently receiving medication and stabilized 1 year; ages 24–50 years	*Intervention:* A supported education program developed by the Occupational Therapy Program at Richard Stockton College called The Bridge Program. The program consisted of weekly sessions for 12 wk. Each session consisted of 2 hr of basic academic skills training, including time management, stress management, study skills, reading, writing, computer, social skills, and exploration of educational/vocational interests; followed by 1 hr of mentoring with an occupational therapy student. *Outcome Measures:* ■ Pre- and posttests for each academic module; Participants Comfort With the Student Role Scale ■ Participant Overall Satisfaction Scale ■ Task Skills (TSS) ■ Interpersonal Skills (ISS) ■ School Behavior Scales ■ Percentage of participants who successfully completed and enrolled in further academic coursework, completed a GED, or obtained employment	Significant improvements were reported on the posttests for 10 of the academic modules. The Participants Comfort with the Student Role Scale indicated more confidence in academic skills and ability to interact with peers/instructors. Significant improvements in scores were noted on the TSS, ISS, and School Behavior Scales. Of the 18 participants, 16 completed the program, and 12 enrolled in further coursework.	Lack of established reliability and validity for outcome assessments. Lack of control group. Small sample size.
Hutchinson, Anthony, Massaro, & Rogers (2007)	Evaluate the success of a supported education/supported employment program for persons with psychiatric disabilities	III—Pretest/posttest N = 61 Mean age: 34.78 years Diagnoses included schizophrenia and depression	*Intervention:* Training for the Future (TFTF), a combined supported education and supported employment program at Boston University's Center for Psychiatric Rehabilitation. The goals of the program are to teach computer skills and recovery coping strategies along with supported employment. A 10-month classroom phase (4 days/wk from 9:30–3:15) consisted of morning instruction computer skills, afternoon practicum time, and the Recovery Workshop. A 2-month 20-hr/wk unpaid internship followed. Upon completion of the internship, students were provided job development and employment support once work was secured. *Outcome Measures:* ■ Ongoing Client Instrument, Empowerment Scale ■ Tennessee Self-Concept Scale ■ Katz Adjustment Scale ■ Client Satisfaction Scale	Overall, there was a positive change in work status. The number of participants working and the number of hours worked per week increased. There was a significant decrease over time in mental health and rehabilitation services use, significant increases in independent living, and positive gains in self-esteem. There were no significant improvements over time on the Katz subscales, but there were improvements in the Total Empowerment scale. Participants reported overall satisfaction with the program.	Lack of control group. Sample selected was highly educated and mostly White and already living independently. Missing long-term data due to dropouts.

Author/Year	Study Objectives	Level/Design & N	Intervention and Outcome Measures	Results	Study Limitations
Lysaker, Bell, & Bioty (1995)	Examine the relationship between measures of cognitive function collected at intake and symptom level measured after 5 months of work rehabilitation	III—Pretest/posttest *N* = 60; 56 male, 4 female	*Intervention:* Participants worked up to 20 hr/wk over 17 wk and attended weekly 50-min group meetings that focused on work experience and offered job-related problem solving and support. *Outcome Measures:* ▪ Positive and Negative Syndrome Scale (PANSS) ▪ Wisconsin Card Sorting Test (WCST) ▪ Gotham Proverbs Test	Total PANSS scores significantly declined after 5 months of work rehabilitation. Results supported the hypothesis that cognitive impairments are associated with a reduction in the clinical effects of work rehabilitation. The WCST and Gotham Proverbs Test were able to correctly classify 83% of participants as improved or unimproved on total symptoms after rehabilitation.	Lack of control group. The analyses were correlational, so causal relationships between cognitive deficits and symptom change could not be determined. The majority of the study population was middle-aged men; results for women or younger men may differ. The work rehabilitation took place only at the VA medical center. It is possible that participants experienced a lesser degree of improved symptoms because they failed to take their medications regularly.
Phelan, Lee, Howe, & Walter (2006)	Describe a pilot group program for parents with a mental illness (Australia)	III—Pretest/posttest *N* = 19 parents completed from 29 participating in the program	*Intervention:* Parenting and Mental Illness Group Program consisted of a 6-wk group program followed by 4 individual follow-up sessions. Interviews at intake. *Outcome Measures:* ▪ Eyberg Child Behaviour Inventory ▪ Parenting Scale	At posttest, 40% fewer parents were in the "intensity" clinical range and 57% fewer in "problem" on Eyberg. On the parenting scale, 26% fewer were in the clinical range for laxness, 45% for overreactivity, and 33% for verbosity.	Small sample size; attrition in program completion and completion of posttest; no comparison statistics were included.

Note. DSM–IV = *Diagnostic and Statistical Manual of Mental Disorders, 4th Edition;* IADLs = instrumental activities of daily living; UCLA = University of California, Los Angeles; UCSD = University of California at San Diego.

Appendix D.
Resources for Recovery-Oriented Practice

American Occupational Therapy Association

- *Occupational Therapy in Mental Health: Considerations for Advanced Practice* (Self-Paced Clinical Course/text)
  http://www.aota.org/CE/SPCC.aspx

National Association of State Mental Health Program Directors

- *Implementing Recovery-Based Care: Tangible Guidance for SMHA*
  http://www.nasmhpd.org/general_files/publications/special%20e-reports/01-fall-04/Report%20Intro.pdf
- *Mental Health Recovery: What Helps and What Hinders*
  http://www.nasmhpd.org/general_files/publications/ntac_pubs/reports/MHSIPReport.pdf
- *Six Core Strategies to Reduce the Use of Seclusion and Restraining Planning Tool*
  http://www.nasmhpd.org/general_files/publications/ntac_pubs/SR%20Plan%20Template%20with%20cover%20
  7-05.pdf
- *Obesity Reduction and Prevention Strategies for Individuals With Serious Mental Illness*
  http://www.nasmhpd.org/general_files/Obesity%2010-8-08.pdf

National Empowerment Center

http://www.power2u.org/

Substance Abuse and Mental Health Services Administration

- National Registry of Evidence-Based Programs and Practices
  http://www.nrepp.samhsa.gov/
- Evidence-Based Practice Tool Kits
  http://www.samhsa.gov/newsroom/advisories/1004145809.aspx
- National Consensus Statement on Mental Health Recovery
  http://store.samhsa.gov/product/SMA05-4129
- *Achieving the Promise: Transforming Mental Health Care in America, Executive Summary* (President's New
  Freedom Commission)
  http://store.samhsa.gov/product/SMA03-3831
- *The 10 By 10 Campaign: A National Wellness Action Plan to Improve Life Expectancy by 10 Years in 10 Years for
  People with Mental Illness*
  http://store.samhsa.gov/product/SMA10-4476

Appendix E.
Selected *Current Procedural Terminology*™ Codes for Occupational Therapy Evaluations and Interventions for Clients With Serious Mental Health Illness

The following chart can guide making clinically appropriate decisions in selecting the most relevant *CPT* code to describe occupational therapy evaluation and intervention for clients with serious mental health illness. Occupational therapy practitioners should use the most appropriate code from the current *CPT* manual based on specific services provided, individual patient goals, payer policy, and common usage.

Examples of Occupational Therapy Evaluation and Intervention	Suggested *CPT* Code(s)
Evaluation	
▪ Evaluate/assess client's overall physical and mental condition through data gathering from multiple sources, including referral source, occupational profile, interview, performance.	**97003**—Occupational therapy evaluation **97004**—Occupational therapy reevaluation
▪ Administer, interpret, and report findings from specific standardized assessments deemed appropriate on the basis of the results of the evaluation process. Examples of common assessments used by the occupational therapist for this population can be found in Table 1 of the main document.	**96125**- Standardized cognitive performance testing (e.g., Ross Information Processing Assessment) per hour of a qualified health care professional's time, both face-to-face time administering tests to the patient and time interpreting these test results and preparing the report
▪ Participate in a team conference as part of a diagnostic team in which the team members convey evaluation findings, diagnoses, and recommendations to a client's family.	**99366**—Medical team conference with an interdisciplinary team of health care professionals, face-to-face with patient and/or family, 30 minutes or more, participation by non-physician qualified health care professional
▪ Participate in a team conference as part of a diagnostic team in which the team members review evaluation findings and clarify diagnostic considerations and recommendations prior to meeting with a client's family.	**99368**—Medical team conference with an interdisciplinary team of health care professionals, patient and/or family not present, 30 minutes or more, participation by non-physician qualified health care professional
Intervention	
▪ Design and have the client train in a daily aerobic exercise program to be completed at home or another venue (e.g., YMCA, swimming pool).	**97110**—Therapeutic procedure, one or more areas, each 15 minutes; therapeutic exercises to develop strength and endurance, range of motion, and flexibility **97113**—Aquatic therapy with therapeutic exercises

(continued)

Examples of Occupational Therapy Evaluation and Intervention	Suggested *CPT* Code(s)
Intervention (continued)	
▪ Develop a "sensory kit" to modulate emotion dysregulation within a specific sensory system. ▪ Train client in use of sensory stimulation to effect change in performance (e.g., being on time for appointments, waking up).	**97112**—Therapeutic procedure, one or more areas, each 15 minutes; neuro-muscular reeducation of movement, balance, coordination, kinesthetic sense, posture, and/or proprioception for sitting and /or standing activities
▪ Develop and train client in the use of occupation-based activities to reduce stress and increase ability to perform avocational or work tasks.	**97530**—Therapeutic activities, direct one-on-one patient contact by the provider (use of dynamic activities to improve functional performance), each 15 minutes
▪ Train client in the use of memory exercises to enhance the ability to remember telephone numbers and e-mail addresses while at home or work.	**97532**—Development of cognitive skills to improve attention, memory, problem solving (includes compensatory training), direct (one-on-one) patient contact by the provider, each 15 minutes
▪ Develop methods (e.g., using alarm clock or phone) to provide alert to take medication. ▪ Develop compensatory strategies and schedules to ensure safe completion of daily personal and household activities (e.g., bathing, meal preparation, washing clothes, household cleaning). ▪ Teach client coping skills to facilitate performance of daily activities. ▪ Train client in methods of adapting environments, habits, and routines to improve specific areas of occupations/activities (e.g., activities of daily living, sleep, meal preparation, hygiene).	**97535**—Self-care and home management training (e.g., activities of daily living and compensatory training, meal preparation, safety procedures, and instruction in use of assistive technology devices/adaptive equipment), direct one-on-one contact by the provider, each 15 minutes
▪ Teach client skills for using public transportation. ▪ Design training program to improve client's social skills while engaging in community activities (e.g., shopping)	**97537**—Community/work reintegration training (e.g., shopping, transportation, money management, avocational activities and/or work environment/modification analysis, work task analysis, use of assistive technology device/adaptive equipment), direct one-on-one contact by the provider, each 15 minutes
▪ Direct a group cognitive remediation program focused on social skills development.	**97150**—Therapeutic procedure(s), group (2 or more individuals; report 97150 for each member of group); group therapy procedures involve constant attendance of the physician or therapist, but by definition do not require one-on-one patient contact by the physician or therapist

Note. The *CPT* 2012 codes referenced in this document do not represent all of the possible codes that may be used in occupational therapy evaluation and intervention. Not all payers will reimburse for all codes. Refer to *CPT 2012* for the complete list of available codes.

CPT[TM] is a trademark of the American Medical Association (AMA). All rights reserved.

Codes shown refer to *CPT 2012. CPT* codes are updated annually. New and revised codes become effective January 1. Always refer to annual updated *CPT* publication for most current codes.

References

Accreditation Council for Occupational Therapy Education. (2012a). Accreditation standards for a doctoral-degree-level educational program for the occupational therapist. *American Journal of Occupational Therapy, 66.*

Accreditation Council for Occupational Therapy Education. (2012b). Accreditation standards for a master's-degree-level educational program for the occupational therapist. *American Journal of Occupational Therapy, 66.*

Accreditation Council for Occupational Therapy Education. (2012c). Accreditation standards for an educational program for the occupational therapy assistant. *American Journal of Occupational Therapy, 66.*

Agency for Healthcare Research and Quality, U.S. Preventive Services Task Force. (2009). *Standard recommendation language.* Retrieved February 14, 2009, from http://www.ahrq.gov/clinic/uspstf/standard.htm

Ali, A. (2009). Disability in schizophrenia and its relation with duration of illness and age of onset. *International Journal of Psychosocial Rehabilitation, 14,* 37–41.

Allen, C. A., Austen, S. K., David, S. K., Earhart, C. A., McCraith, D. B., & Williams, L. R. (2007). *Manual for the Allen Cognitive Level Screen–5 and Large Cognitive Level Screen–5.* Colchester, CT: S&S Worldwide.

Allen, C. K., Earhart, C. A., & Blue, T. (1992). *Occupational therapy treatment goals for the physically and cognitively disabled.* Bethesda, MD: American Occupational Therapy Association.

American Medical Association. (2011). *CPT 2012.* Chicago: Author.

American Occupational Therapy Association. (1979). *Occupational therapy product output reporting system and uniform terminology for reporting occupational therapy services.* (Available from the American Occupational Therapy Association, 4720 Montgomery Lane, P.O. Box 31220, Bethesda, MD 20824–1220.)

American Occupational Therapy Association. (1989). *Uniform terminology for occupational therapy* (2nd ed.). (Available from the American Occupational Therapy Association, 4720 Montgomery Lane, P.O. Box 31220, Bethesda, MD 20824–1220)

American Occupational Therapy Association. (1994). Uniform terminology for occupational therapy (3rd ed.). *American Journal of Occupational Therapy, 48,* 1047–1054.

American Occupational Therapy Association. (2002). Occupational therapy practice framework: Domain and process. *American Journal of Occupational Therapy, 56,* 609–639.

American Occupational Therapy Association. (2006). Policy 1.44: Categories of occupational therapy personnel. In *Policy manual* (2011 ed., pp. 33–34). Bethesda, MD: Author.

American Occupational Therapy Association. (2007). AOTA's *Centennial Vision* and executive summary. *American Journal of Occupational Therapy, 61,* 613–614.

American Occupational Therapy Association. (2008a). Guidelines for documentation of occupational therapy. *American Journal of Occupational Therapy, 62,* 684–690.

American Occupational Therapy Association. (2008b). Occupational therapy practice framework: Domain and process (2nd ed.). *American Journal of Occupational Therapy, 62,* 625–683.

American Occupational Therapy Association. (2009). Guidelines for supervision, roles, and responsibilities during the delivery of occupational therapy services. *American Journal of Occupational Therapy, 63,* 797–803.

American Occupational Therapy Association. (2010). Standards of practice for occupational therapy. *American Journal of Occupational Therapy, 64,* S106–S111.

American Psychiatric Association. (2000). *Diagnostic and statistical manual of mental disorders* (4th ed., text rev.). Washington, DC: Author.

Anzai, N., Yoneda, S., Kumagai, N., Nakamura, Y., Ikebuchi, E., & Liberman, R. P. (2002). Training persons with schizophrenia in illness self-management: A randomized controlled trial in Japan. *Psychiatric Services, 53,* 545–547.

Bartels, S. J., Forester, B., Mueser, K. T., Miles, K. M., Dums, A. R., Pratt, S. I., & Perkins, L. (2004). Enhanced skills training and health care management for older persons with severe mental illness. *Community Mental Health Journal, 40,* 75–90.

Baum, C., Morrison, T., Hahn, M., & Edwards, D. (2003). *Executive Function Performance Test: Test protocol booklet.* St. Louis, MO: Washington University, School of Medicine.

Beard, J. G., & Ragheb, M. G. (1980). The Leisure Satisfaction Scale. *Journal of Leisure Research, 12,* 20–33.

Becker, P. (2006). Treatment of sleep dysfunction and psychiatric disorders. *Current Treatment Options in Neurology, 8,* 367–375.

Bell, M. D., & Bryson, G. (2003). Work rehabilitation in schizophrenia: Does cognitive impairment limit improvement? *Schizophrenia Bulletin, 27,* 269–279.

Bell, M., Bryson, G., Greig, T., Corcoran, C., & Wexler, B. E. (2001). Neurocognitive enhancement therapy with work therapy: Effects on neuropsychological test performance. *Archives of General Psychiatry, 58,* 763–768.

Bell, M. D., Fiszdon, J. M., Greig, T. C., & Bryson, G. J. (2005). Can older people with schizophrenia benefit from work rehabilitation? *Journal of Nervous and Mental Disease, 193,* 293–301.

Bell, M., Lysaker, P., & Bryson, G. (2003). A behavioral intervention to improve work performance in schizophrenia: Work Behavior Inventory feedback. *Journal of Vocational Rehabilitation, 18,* 43–50.

Bellack, A. S. (2004). Skills training for people with severe mental illness. *Psychiatric Rehabilitation Journal, 27,* 375–391.

Beynon, S., Soares-Weiser, K., Woolacott, N., Duffy, S., & Geddes, J. R. (2008). Psychosocial interventions for the prevention of relapse in bipolar disorder: Systematic review of controlled trials. *British Journal of Psychiatry, 192,* 5–10.

Bickes, M. B., DeLoache, S. N., Dicer, J. R., & Miller, S. C. (2001). Effectiveness of experiential and verbal occupational therapy groups in a community mental health setting. *Occupational Therapy in Mental Health, 17,* 51–72.

Bond, G. R. (2004). Supported employment: Evidence for an evidence-based practice. *Psychiatric Rehabilitation Journal, 27,* 345–356.

Bond, G. R., Drake, R. E., & Becker, D. R. (2008). An update on randomized controlled trials of evidence-based supported employment. *Psychiatric Rehabilitation Journal, 31,* 280–290.

Bottlender, R., Strauss, A., & Möller, H. J. (2010). Social disability in schizophrenia, schizoaffective disorder, and affective disorders: 15 years after first admission. *Schizophrenia Research, 116,* 9–15.

Braveman, B., Robson, M., Velozo, C., Kielhofner, G., Fisher, G., Forsyth, K., & Kerschbaum, J. (2005). *A user's guide to the Worker Role Interview (Version 10.0)*. Chicago: Model of Human Occupation Clearinghouse, University of Illinois at Chicago.

Brayman, S. J., Kirby, T. F., Misenheimer, A. M., & Short, M.J. (1976). Comprehensive Occupational Therapy Evaluation Scale. *American Journal of Occupational Therapy, 30*, 94–100.

Briand, C., Vasiliadis, H. M., Lesage, A., Lalonde, P., Stip, E., Nicole, L., Reinharz, D., ... Villeneuve, K. (2006). Including integrated psychological treatment as part of standard medical therapy for patients with schizophrenia: Clinical outcomes. *Journal of Nervous and Mental Disease, 194*, 463–470.

Brown, C., Cromwell, R. L., Filion, D., Dunn, W., & Tollefson, N. (2002). Sensory processing in schizophrenia: Missing and avoiding information. *Schizophrenia Research, 55*, 187–195.

Brown, C., & Dunn, W. (2002). *Adolescent/Adult Sensory Profile*. San Antonio, TX: Psychological Corporation.

Brown, C., Goetz, J., Van Sciver A., Sullivan, D., & Hamera, E. (2006). A psychiatric rehabilitation approach to weight loss. *Psychiatric Rehabilitation Journal, 29*, 267–273.

Brown, C., Moyers, P., Sells, C., Learnard, L., Mahaffey, L. M., Pitts, D. B., et al. (2006). *Report of Ad Hoc Committee on Mental Health Practice in Occupational Therapy*. Retrieved from http://www.aota.org/News/Centennial/Background/AdHoc/2006/40406.aspx?FT=.pdf

Brown, C., Rempfer, M., & Hamera, E. (2002). Teaching grocery shopping skills to people with schizophrenia. *Occupational Therapy Journal of Research: Occupation, Participation and Health, 22*(Suppl. 1), 90S–91S.

Brown, C., Rempfer, M., & Hamera, E. (2009). *Test of Grocery Shopping Skills*. Bethesda, MD: AOTA Press.

Bryson, G., Bell, M. D., Lysaker, P., & Zito, W. (1997). The Work Behavior Inventory: A scale for the assessment of work behavior for people with severe mental illness. *Psychiatric Rehabilitation Journal, 20*, 47–55.

Buchain, P. C., Vizzotto, A. D., Henna Neto, J., & Elkis, H. (2003). Randomized controlled trial of occupational therapy in patients with treatment-resistant schizophrenia. *Revista Brasileira de Psiquiatria, 25*, 26–30.

Bussema, E. F., & Bussema, K. E. (2007). Gilead revisited: Faith and recovery. *Psychiatric Rehabilitation Journal, 30*, 301–305.

Bybee, D., Mowbray, C. T., Oyserman, D., & Lewandowski, L. (2003). Variability in community functioning of mothers with serious mental illness. *Journal of Behavioral Health Services and Research, 30*, 269–289.

Cabassa, L. J., Ezell, J. M., & Lewis-Fernandez, R. (2010). Lifestyle interventions for adults with serious mental illness: A systematic literature review. *Psychiatric Services, 61*, 774–782.

Chafetz, L., White, M., Collins-Bride, G., Cooper, B. A., & Nickens, J. (2008). Clinical trial of wellness training: Health promotion for severely mentally ill adults. *Journal of Nervous and Mental Disease, 196*, 475–483.

Champagne, T., & Stromberg, N. (2004). Sensory approaches in inpatient psychiatric settings: Innovative alternatives to seclusion and restraint. *Journal of Psychosocial Nursing and Mental Health Services, 42*, 34–35.

Chan, S. H., Lee, S. W., & Chan, I. W. (2007). TRIP: A psycho-educational programme in Hong Kong for people with schizophrenia. *Occupational Therapy International, 14*, 86–98.

Chern, J., Kielhofner, G., de las Heras, C., & Magalhaes, L. (1996). The Volitional Questionnaire: Psychometric development and practical use. *American Journal of Occupational Therapy, 50,* 516–525.

Choi, K. H., & Kwon, J. H. (2006). Social cognition enhancement training for schizophrenia: A preliminary randomized controlled trial. *Community Mental Health Journal, 42,* 177–187.

Collins, M. E., Bybee, D., & Mowbray, C. T. (1998). Effectiveness of supported education for individuals with psychiatric disabilities: Results from an experimental study. *Community Mental Health Journal, 34,* 595–613.

Colton, C. W., & Manderscheid, R. W. (2006). Congruencies in increased mortality rates, years of potential life lost, and causes of death among public mental health clients in eight states. *Preventing Chronic Disease, 3,* 1–14.

Cook, J. A. (2006). Employment barriers for persons with psychiatric disabilities: Update of a report for the President's Commission. *Psychiatric Services, 57,* 1391–1405.

Cook, J. A., Copeland, M. E., Corey, L. Buffington, E., Jonikas, J. A., & Curtis, L. C. (2010). Developing the evidence base for peerled services: Changes among participants following Wellness Recovery Action Planning (WRAP) Education in two statewide initiatives. *Psychiatric Rehabilitation Journal, 34,* 113–120.

Cook, J. A., Leff, H. S., Blyler, C. R., Gold, P. B., Goldberg, R. W., Mueser, K. T., ... Burke-Miller, J. (2005). Results of a multisite randomized trial of supported employment interventions for individuals with severe mental illness. *Archives of General Psychiatry, 62,* 505–512.

Cook, J. A., Lehman, A. F., Drake, R., McFarlane, W. R., Gold, P. B., Leff, H. S., ... Grey, D. D. (2005). Integration of psychiatric and vocational services: A multisite randomized, controlled trial of supported

employment. *American Journal of Psychiatry, 162,* 1948–1956.

Cook, S., Chambers, E., & Coleman, J. H. (2009). Occupational therapy for people with psychotic conditions in community settings: A pilot randomized controlled trial. *Clinical Rehabilitation, 23,* 40–52.

Corrigan, P. W. (1991). Social skills training in adult psychiatric populations: A meta-analysis. *Journal of Behavior Therapy and Experimental Psychiatry, 22,* 203–210.

Couture, S. M., Penn, D. L., & Roberts, D. L. (2006). The functional significance of social cognition in schizophrenia: A review. *Schizophrenia Bulletin, 32*(Suppl. 1), S44–S63.

Crowther, R. E., Marshall, M., Bond, G. R., & Huxley, P. (2001). Helping people with severe mental illness to obtain work: Systematic review. *British Medical Journal, 322,* 204–208.

Dilk, M. N., & Bond, G. R. (1996). Meta-analytic evaluation of skills training research for individuals with severe mental illness. *Journal of Consulting and Clinical Psychology, 64,* 1337–1345.

Dixon, L. B., Dickerson, F., Bellack, A. S., Bennett, M., Dickerson, D., Goldberg, R. W., & Schizophrenia Patient Outcomes Research Team. (2010). The 2009 schizophrenia PORT psychosocial treatment recommendations and summary statements. *Schizophrenia Bulletin, 36,* 48–70.

Draine, J., Salzer, M. S., Culhane, D. P., & Hadley, T. R. (2002). Role of social disadvantage in crime, joblessness, and homelessness among persons with serious mental illness. *Psychiatric Services, 53,* 565–573.

Duncombe, L. W. (2004). Comparing learning of cooking in home and clinic for people with schizophrenia. *American Journal of Occupational Therapy, 58,* 272–278.

Dunlop, D. D., Manheim, L. M., Song, J., Lyons, J. S., & Chang, R. W. (2005). Incidence of disability among preretirement adults: The impact of depression. *American Journal of Public Health, 95,* 2003–2008.

Dunn, A. L., Trivedi, M. H., Kampert, J. B., Clark, C. G., & Chambliss, H. O. (2005). Exercise treatment for depression. *American Journal of Preventive Medicine, 28,* 1–8.

Dunn, A. L., Trivedi, M. H., & O'Neal, H. A. (2001). Physical activity dose–response effects on outcomes of depression and anxiety. *Medicine and Science in Sports and Exercise, 33*(6, Suppl.), S587–S597.

Dunn, W., McClain, L. H., Brown, C., & Youngstrom, M. J. (1998). The ecology of human performance. In M. E. Neistadt & E. B. Crepeau (Eds.), *Willard and Spackman's occupational therapy* (9th ed., pp. 525–535). Philadelphia: Lippincott Williams & Wilkins.

Edgelow, M., & Krupa, T. (2011). Randomized controlled pilot study of an occupational time-use intervention for people with serious mental illness. *American Journal of Occupational Therapy, 65,* 267–276.

Eklund, M. (2001). Psychiatric patients' occupational roles: Changes over time and associations with self-rated quality of life. *Scandinavian Journal of Occupational Therapy, 8,* 125–130.

Eklund, M., & Leufstadius, C. (2007). Occupational factors and aspects of health and well-being in individuals with persistent mental illness living in the community. *Canadian Journal of Occupational Therapy, 74,* 303–313.

Endicott, J., Spitzer, R. L., Fleiss, J. L., & Cohen, J. (1976). The Global Assessment Scale: A procedure for measuring overall severity of psychiatric disturbance. *Archives of General Psychiatry, 33,* 766–771.

Ennals, P., & Fossey, E. (2007). The Occupational Performance History Instrument in community mental health case management: Consumer and occupational therapy perspectives. *Australian Occupational Therapy Journal, 54,* 11–21.

Epstein, J., Barker, P., Vorburger, M., & Murtha, C. (2002). *Serious mental illness and its co-occurrence with substance use disorders.* A report of the Department of Health & Human Services (Section 1.2). Rockville, MD: Substance Abuse and Mental Health Services Administration.

Fisher, A. G. (2001). *Assessment of Motor and Process Skills, Vol. 2: User manual* (4th ed.). Fort Collins, CO: Three Star Press.

Folkman, S., & Lazarus, R. W. (1988). *Manual for the Ways of Coping Questionnaire.* Palo Alto, CA: Consulting Psychologists Press.

Forsyth, K., Deshpande, S., Kielhofner, G., Henriksoon, C., Haglund, L., Olson, L., & Supriya, K. (2005). *Occupational Circumstances Assessment Interview Rating Scale* (Version 4.0). Chicago: Model of Human Occupation Clearinghouse, University of Illinois at Chicago.

Forsyth, K., Salamy, M., Simon, S., & Kielhofner, G. (1998). *The Assessment of Communication and Interaction Skills* (Version 4.0). Chicago: Department of Occupational Therapy, University of Illinois at Chicago.

Frank, E., Kupfer, D. J., Thase, M. E., Mallinger, A. G., Swartz, H. A., Faglioni, A. M., ... Monk, T. (2005). Two-year outcomes for interpersonal and social rhythm therapy for individuals with bipolar I disorder. *Archives of General Psychiatry, 62,* 996–1004.

Frank, E., Soreca, I, Swartz, H. A., Fagiolini, A. M., Mallinger, A. G., Thase, M. E., ... Kupfer, D. J. (2008). The role of interpersonal and social rhythm therapy in improving occupational functioning in patients with bipolar I disorder. *American Journal of Psychiatry, 165,* 1559–1565.

Furukawa, T. A., Takeuchi, H., Hiroe, T., Mashiko, H., Kamei, K., Kitamura, T., & Takahashi, K. (2010). Symptomatic recovery and social functioning in major depression. *Acta Psychiatrica Scandinavica, 103,* 257–261.

Gioia, D. (2005). Career development in schizophrenia: A heuristic framework. *Community Mental Health Journal, 41,* 307–325.

Glynn, S. M., Marder, S. R., Liberman, R. P., Blair, K., Wirshing, W. C., Wirshing, D. A, & Mintz, J. (2002). Supplementing clinic-based skills training with manual-based community support sessions: Effects on social adjustment of patients with schizophrenia. *American Journal of Psychiatry, 159,* 829–837.

Gold, P. B., Meisler, N., Santos, A. B., Carnemolla, M. A., Williams, O. H., & Keleher, J. (2006). Randomized trial of supported employment integrated with assertive community treatment for rural adults with severe mental illness. *Schizophrenia Bulletin, 32,* 378–395.

Granholm, E., McQuaid, J. R., McClure, F. S., Auslander, L. A., Perivoliotis, D., Pedrelli, P., & Jeste, D. V. (2005). A randomized, controlled trial of cognitive behavioral social skills training for middle-aged and older outpatients with chronic schizophrenia. *American Journal of Psychiatry, 162,* 520–529.

Grawe, R. W., Falloon, I. R. H., Widen, J. H., & Skogvoll, E. (2006). Two years of continued early treatment for recent-onset schizophrenia: A randomised controlled study. *Acta Psychiatrica Scandinavica, 114,* 328–36.

Green, M. F. (2006). Cognitive impairment and functional outcome in schizophrenia and bipolar disorder. *Journal of Clinical Psychiatry, 62*(Suppl. 9), 3–8.

Gualtieri, C. T., Johnson, L. G., & Benedict, K. B. (2006). Neurocognition in depression: Patients on and off medication versus healthy comparison subjects. *Journal of Neuropsychiatry and Clinical Neuroscience, 18,* 217–225.

Gutman, S. A., Kerner, R., Zombek, I., Dulek, J., & Ramsey, C. A. (2009). Supported education for adults with psychiatric disabilities: Effectiveness of an occupational therapy program. *American Journal of Occupational Therapy, 63,* 245–254.

Gutman, S. A., Schindler, V. P., Furphy, K. A., Klein, K., Lisak, J. M., & Durham, D. P. (2007). The effectiveness of a supported education program for adults with psychiatric disabilities: The Bridge Program. *Occupational Therapy in Mental Health, 23,* 21–38.

Hadas-Lidor, N., Katz, N., Tyano, S., & Weizman, A. (2001). Effectiveness of dynamic cognitive intervention in rehabilitation of clients with schizophrenia. *Clinical Rehabilitation, 15,* 349–359.

Halford, W. K., Harrison, C., Kalyansundaram Moutrey, C., & Simpson, S. (1995). Preliminary results from a psychoeducation program to rehabilitate chronic patients. *Psychiatric Services, 46,* 1189–1191.

Harvey, P. D., Velligan, D. I., & Bellack, A. S. (2007). Performance based measures of functional skills: Usefulness in clinical treatment studies. *Schizophrenia Bulletin, 33,* 1138–1148.

Helfrich, C. A., Aviles, A. M., Badiani, C., Walens, D., & Sabol, P. (2006). Life skill interventions with homeless youth, domestic violence victims, and adults with mental illness. *Occupational Therapy in Health Care, 20,* 189–207.

Helfrich, C. A., Chan, D. V., & Sabol, P. (2011). Cognitive predictors of life skill intervention outcomes for adults with mental illness at risk for homelessness. *American Journal of Occupational Therapy, 65,* 277–286. doi:10.5014/ajot.2011.001321

Henry, J. D., Green, M. J., de Lucia, A., Restuccia, C., McDonald, S., & O'Donnell, M. (2007). Emotional dysregulation in schizophrenia: Reduced amplification of emotional expression is associated with emotional blunting. *Schizophrenia Research, 95,* 197–204.

Holland, J. L. (1997). *Making vocational choices: A theory of vocational personalities and work environments* (3rd ed.). Odessa, FL: Psychological Assessment Resources.

Holm, M. B., & Rogers, J. C. (1999). Performance Assessment of Self Care Skills. In B. J. Hemphill-Pearson (Ed.), *Assessment in occupational therapy mental health* (pp. 117–124). Thorofare, NJ: Slack.

Honey, A. (2003). The impact of mental illness on employment: Consumers' perspectives. *Work, 20,* 267–276.

Huckshorn, K. A. (2005). *Six core strategies to reduce the use of seclusion and restraint planning tool.* Alexandria, VA: National Association of State Mental Health Program Directors.

Hutchinson, D., Anthony, W., Massaro, J., & Rogers, E. S. (2007). Evaluation of a combined supported computer education and employment training program for persons with psychiatric disabilities. *Psychiatric Rehabilitation Journal, 30,* 189–197.

Hutchinson, D. S., Skrinar, G. S., & Cross, C. (1999). The role of improved physical fitness in rehabilitation and recovery. *Psychiatric Rehabilitation Journal, 22,* 355–359.

Iwama, M. K. (2005). The *kawa* (river) model: Nature, life, flow, and the power of culturally relevant occupational therapy. In F. Kronenberg, S. Algado, & N. Pollard (Eds.), *Occupational therapy without borders: Learning from the spirit of survivors* (pp. 213–237). Edinburgh, UK: Elsevier/Churchill Livingstone.

Jenkinson, N., Ownsworth, T., & Shum, D. (2007). Utility of the Canadian Occupational Performance Measure in community-based brain injury rehabilitation. *Brain Injury, 21,* 1283–1294.

Kates, N., Nikolaou, L., Ballie, B., & Hess, J. (1997). An in-home employment program for people with mental illness. *Psychiatric Rehabilitation Journal, 20,* 56–61.

Katz, N., Itzkovich, M., Averbuch, S., & Elazar, B. (1989). Loewenstein Occupational Therapy Cognitive Assessment (LOTCA) Battery for brain-injured Patients: Reliability and validity. *American Journal of Occupational Therapy, 43,* 184–192.

Kay, S. R., Fisbein, A., & Opler, C.A. (1987). Positive and negative syndrome scale (PANSS) for schizophrenia. *Schizophrenia Bulletin, 13,* 261–276

Keefe, R. S., Poe, M., Walker, T. M., Kang, J. W., & Harvey, P. D. (2006). The Schizophrenia Cognition Rating Scale SCoRS: Interview-based assessment and its relationship to cognition, real world functioning and functional capacity. *American Journal of Psychiatry, 163,* 426–432.

Kelley, M. P., Coursey, R. D., & Selby, P. M. (1997). Therapeutic adventures outdoors: A demonstration of benefits for people with mental illness. *Psychiatric Rehabilitation Journal, 20,* 61–73.

Kern, R. S., Green, M. F., Mintz, J., & Liberman, R. (2003). Does "errorless learning" compensate for neuro-cognitive impairments in work rehabilitation of persons with schizophrenia? *Psychological Medicine, 33,* 443–452.

Kern, R. S., Glynn, S. M., Horan, W. P., & Marder, S. R. (2009). Psychosocial treatments to promote functional recovery in schizophrenia. *Schizophrenia Bulletin, 35,* 347–361.

Kern, R. S., Liberman, R. P., Kopelowicz, A., Mintz, J., & Green, M. F. (2002). Application of errorless learning for improving work performance in persons with schizophrenia. *American Journal of Psychiatry, 159,* 1921–1926.

Kielhofner, G., & Brinson, M. (1989). Development and evaluation of an aftercare program for young chronic psychiatrically disabled adults. *Occupational Therapy in Mental Health, 9*(2), 1–25.

Kielhofner, G., Mallinson, T., Crawford, C., Nowak, M., Rigby, M., Henry, A., & Walens, D. (2004). *A user's manual for the Occupational Performance History Interview* (Version 2.1). Chicago: Model of Human Occupation Clearinghouse, University of Illinois at Chicago.

Kielhofner, G., & Neville, A. (1983). *The Modified Interest Checklist*. Chicago: Model of Human Occupation Clearinghouse, University of Illinois at Chicago.

Kopelowicz, A., Liberman, R. P., Wallace, C. J., Aguirre, F., & Mintz, J. (2006). Differential performance of job skills in schizophrenia: An experimental analysis. *Journal of Rehabilitation, 72,* 31–39.

Kopelowicz, A., Wallace, C. J., & Zarate, R. (1998). Teaching psychiatric inpatients to re-enter the community: A brief method of improving the continuity of care. *Psychiatric Services, 49,* 1313–1316.

Kopelowicz, A., Zarate, R., Gonzalez Smith, V., Mintz, J., & Liberman, R. P. (2003). Disease management in Latinos with schizophrenia: A family-assisted, skills training approach. *Schizophrenia Bulletin, 29,* 211–227.

Kurtz, M., Seltzer, J. C., Shagan, D. S., Thime, W. R., & Wexler, B. E. (2007). Computer-assisted cognitive remediation in schizophrenia: What is the active ingredient? *Schizophrenia Research, 89,* 251–260.

Latimer, E. A., Lecomte, T., Becker, D. R., Drake, R. E., Duclos, I., Piat, M., & Xie, H. (2006). Gerneralisability of the individual placement and support model of supported employment: Results of a Canadian randomised controlled trial. *British Journal of Psychiatry, 189,* 65–73.

Law, M., Baptiste, S., Carsell, A., McColl, M. A., Polatajko, H., & Pollock, N. (1998). *The Canadian Occupational Performance Measure* (3rd ed.). Toronto, Ontario: Canadian Occupational Therapy Association.

Law, M., & Baum, C. (1998). Evidence-based occupational therapy. *Canadian Journal of Occupational Therapy, 65,* 131–135.

Leclerc, C., Lesage, A. D., Ricard, N., Lecomte, T., & Cyr, M. (2000). Assessment of a new rehabilitative coping skills module for persons with schizophrenia. *American Journal of Orthopsychiatry, 70,* 380–388.

Lee, H.-L., Tan, H.-K., Ma, H.-I., Tsai, C.-Y., & Liu, Y.-K. (2006). Effectiveness of a work-related stress management program in patients with chronic schizophrenia. *American Occupational Therapy Journal, 60,* 435–441.

Leonardelli, C. (1988). *Milwaukee Evaluation of Daily Living Skills*. Thorofare, NJ: Slack.

Leucht, S., Burkard, T., Henderson, J., Maj, M., & Sartorius, N. (2007). Physical illness and schizophrenia: A review of the literature. *Acta Psychiatrica Scandinavica, 116,* 317–333.

Leufstadius, D., & Eklund, M. (2008). Time use among individuals with persistent mental illness: Identifying risk factors for imbalance in daily activities. *Scandinavian Journal of Occupational Therapy, 15,* 23–33.

Levin, S. J., Like, R. C., & Gottlieb, J. E. (2000). ETHNIC: A framework for culturally competent clinical practice. *Patient Care, 34,* 188–189.

Liberman, R. P., Wallace, C. J., Blackwell, G., Kopelowicz, A., Vaccaro, J. V., & Mintz, J. (1998). Skills training versus psychosocial occupational therapy for persons with persistent schizophrenia. *American Journal of Psychiatry, 155,* 1087–1091.

Lieberman, D., & Scheer, J. (2002). AOTA's evidence-based literature review project: An overview. *American Journal of Occupational Therapy, 56,* 344–349.

Lindenmayer, J. P., McGurk, S. R., Mueser, K. T., Khan, A., Wance, D., Hoffman, L., ... Haiyi, X. (2008). A randomized controlled trial of cognitive remediation among inpatients with persistent mental illness. *Psychiatric Services, 59,* 241–247.

Linkins, K. W., Lucca, A. M., Housman, M., & Smith, S. A. (2006). Use of PASRR programs to assess serious mental illness and service access in nursing homes. *Psychiatric Services, 57,* 325–332.

Lysaker, P., Bell, M., & Bioty, S. (1995). Cognitive deficits in schizophrenia: Prediction of symptom change for participators in work rehabilitation. *Journal of Nervous and Mental Disorders, 5,* 332–336.

Lysaker, P. H., & Buck, K. D. (2007). Neurocognitive deficits as a barrier to psychosocial function in schizophrenia: Effects on learning, coping and self concept. *Journal of Psychosocial Nursing and Mental Health Services, 45,* 24–31.

Malkoff-Schwartz, S., Frank, D., Anderson, B., Sherrill, J. T., Siegel, L., Patterson, D., & Kupfer, D. J. (1998). Stressful life events and social rhythm disruption in the onset of manic and depressive bipolar episodes: A preliminary investigation. *Archives of General Psychiatry, 55,* 702–707.

Marder, S. R., Wirshing, W. C., Mintz, J., McKenzie, J., Johnston, K., Eckman, T. A., ... Liberman, R. P. (1996). Two-year outcome of social skills training and group psychotherapy for outpatients with schizophrenia. *American Journal of Psychiatry, 153,* 1585–1592.

McGrath, J., & Hayes, R. L. (2000). Cognitive rehabilitation for people with schizophrenia and related conditions. *Cochrane Database of Systematic Reviews,* Issue 3, Article No. CD000968. doi:10.1002/14651858.CD000968.

McGurk, S. R., Mueser, K. T., Feldman, K., Wolfe, R., & Pascaris, A. (2007). Cognitive training for supported employment: 2–3 year outcomes of a randomized controlled trial. *American Journal of Psychiatry, 164,* 437–441.

McGurk, S. R., Twamley, E. W., Sitzer, D. I., McHugo, G. J., & Mueser, K. T. (2007). A meta-analysis of cognitive remediation in schizophrenia. *American Journal of Psychiatry, 164,* 1791–1802.

Megivern, D., Pellerito, S., & Mowbray, C. (2003). Barriers to higher education for adults with psychiatric disabilities. *Psychiatric Rehabilitation Journal, 26,* 217–231.

Midorikawa, A., Hashimotor, R., Noguchi, H., Saitoh, O., Kunugi, H., & Nakamura, K. (2008). Impairment of motor dexterity in schizophrenia assessed by a novel finger movement test. *Psychiatry Research, 159,* 281–289.

Mileu, P., Ho, B. C., Arnd, S., & Andreason, N. C. (2005). Predictive values of neurocognition and negative symptoms on functional outcome in schizophrenia: A longitudinal first episode study with 7-year follow up. *American Journal of Psychiatry, 162,* 495–506.

Moore-Corner, R. A., Kielhofner, G., & Olson, L. (1998). *A user's manual for the Work Environment Impact Scale, Version 2.0.* Chicago: Model of Human Occupation Clearinghouse, University of Illinois.

Moos, R. (1994). *Work Environment Scale manual: Development, applications, research* (3rd ed.). Palo Alto, CA: Consulting Psychologists Press.

Moriana, J. A., Alarcon, E., & Herruzo, J. (2006). In-home psychosocial skills training for patients with schizophrenia. *Psychiatric Services, 57,* 260–262.

Mowbray, C. T., Collins, M. E., Bellamy, C. D., Megivern, D. A., Bybee, D., & Szilvagy, S. (2005). Supported education for adults with psychiatric disabilities: An innovation for social work and psychiatric rehabilitation practice. *Social Work, 50,* 7–20.

Moyers, P. A., & Dale, L. M. (2007). *The guide to occupational therapy practice* (2nd ed.). Bethesda, MD: AOTA Press.

Mueser, K. T., Aalto, S., Becker, D. R., Ogden, J. S., Wolfe, R. S., Schiavo, D., et al. (2005). The effectiveness of skills training for improving outcomes in supported employment. *Psychiatric Services, 56,* 1254–1260.

Mueser, K. T., Clark, R. E., Haines, M., Drake, R. E., McHugo, G. J., Bond, G. R., et al. (2004). The Hartford study of supported employment for persons with severe mental illness. *Journal of Consulting and Clinical Psychology, 72,* 479–490.

National Institute of Mental Health. (1987). *Toward a model for a comprehensive community-based mental health system.* Washington, DC: Author.

National Institute of Mental Health. (2010). *The numbers count: Mental disorder in America.* Retrieved January 24, 2012, from http://www.nimh.nih.gov/health/publications/the-numbers-count-mental-disorders-in-america/index.shtml

Neistadt, M. E. (1992). The Rabideau Kitchen Evaluation–Revised: An assessment of meal preparation skill. Occupational Therapy Journal of Research, 12, 242–255.

Newcomer, J. W., & Hennekens, C. H. (2007). Serious mental illness and risk of cardiovascular disease. *Journal of the American Medical Association, 298,* 1794–1796.

New Freedom Commission on Mental Health. (2003). *Achieving the promise: Transforming mental health care in America. Final report* (DHHS Publication No. SMA-03–3832). Rockville, MD: U.S. Department of Health and Human Services.

O'Carrol, R. E., Russell, H. H., Lawrie, S. M., & Johnstone, E. C. (1999). Errorless learning and the cognitive rehabilitation of memory impaired schizophrenic patients. *Psychological Medicine, 29,* 105–112.

O'Connell, M., Tondora, J., Evans, A. C., Croog, G., & Davidson, L. (2005). From rhetoric to routine: Assessing recovery-oriented practices in a state mental health and addiction system. *Psychiatric Rehabilitation Journal, 28,* 378–386.

Patterson, T. L., Bucardo, J., McKibbin, C. L., Mausbach, B. T., Moore, D., Barrio, C., ... Jeste, D. V. (2005). Development and pilot testing of a new psychosocial intervention for older Latinos with chronic psychosis. *Schizophrenia Bulletin, 31,* 922–930.

Patterson, T. L., Goldman, S., McKibbin, C. L., Hughs, T., & Jeste, D. V. (2001). UCSD Performance-Based Skills Assessment: Development of a new measure of everyday functioning for severely mentally ill adults. *Schizophrenia Bulletin, 27,* 235–245.

Patterson, T. L., Mausbach, B. T., McKibbin, C., Goldman, S., Bucardo, J., & Jeste, D. V. (2006). Functional Adaptation Skills Training (FAST): A randomized trial of a psychosocial intervention for middle-aged and older patients with chronic psychotic disorders. *Schizophrenia Research, 86,* 291–299.

Patterson, T. L., McKibbin, C., Taylor, M., Goldman, S., Davila-Fraga, W., Bucardo, J., & Jeste, D. V. (2003). Functional Adaptation Skills Training (FAST): A pilot psychosocial intervention study in middle-aged and older patients with chronic psychotic disorders. *American Journal of Geriatric Psychiatry, 11,* 17–23.

Peck, M. C., & Scheffler, R. M. (2002). An analysis of the definition of mental illness used in state parity laws. *Psychiatric Services, 53,* 1089–1095.

Penn, D. L., Sanna, C. J., & Roberts, D. L. (2008). Social cognition in schizophrenia: An overview. *Schizophrenia Bulletin, 34,* 408–411.

Phelan, R., Lee, L., Howe, D., & Walter, G. (2006). Parenting and mental illness: A pilot group programme for parents. *Australasian Psychiatry, 14,* 399–402.

Phipps, S., & Richardson, P. (2007). Outpatient occupational therapy outcomes for clients with brain injury and stroke using the Canadian Occupational Performance Measure. *American Journal of Occupational Therapy, 61,* 328–334.

Pilling, S., Bebbington, P., Kuipers, E., Garety, P., Geddes, J., Martindale, B., ... Morgan, C. (2002). Psychological treatments in schizophrenia: II. Meta-analyses of randomized controlled trials of social skills training and cognitive remediation. *Psychological Medicine, 32,* 783–791.